Dissociative Retreat and Addiction

Dissociative Retreat and Addiction presents a new theoretical and clinical model for understanding and treating addiction. Giuseppe Craparo examines how addictive behaviours develop as the result of complex psychic and physical conditions, working in conjunction with a specific addictive-object, and explores factors including poor relational and developmental history, strong emotional pain and psychopathological conditions including anxiety, depression, personality disorders and psychosis. Craparo's clinical, developmental–relational model conceptualizes addictive symptoms as reenactments of traumatic memories and observes how addictive-objects are used as defensive somato-psychic retreats from the intense emotions associated with traumatic memories. The book provides a full overview of the model with clinical examples and theoretical underpinnings. *Dissociative Retreat and Addiction* will be of great interest to psychoanalysts, psychotherapists, and other professionals working with addiction and trauma.

Giuseppe Craparo is a psychologist, Psychoanalyst, full professor of Clinical Psychology, and coordinator of the MSc programme in Clinical Psychology at the Kore University of Enna, Italy.

Dissociative Retreat and Addiction

Trauma, Dissociation, and Affect Dysregulation

Giuseppe Craparo

Routledge
Taylor & Francis Group
LONDON AND NEW YORK

Designed cover image: Getty Images

First published 2027
by Routledge
4 Park Square, Milton Park, Abingdon, Oxon OX14 4RN

and by Routledge
605 Third Avenue, New York, NY 10158

Routledge is an imprint of the Taylor & Francis Group, an Informa business

British Library Cataloguing-in-Publication Data
A catalogue record for this book is available from the British Library

ISBN: 978-1-032-35106-3 (hbk)
ISBN: 978-1-032-35105-6 (pbk)
ISBN: 978-1-003-32531-4 (ebk)

DOI: 10.4324/9781003325314

Typeset in Times New Roman
by Taylor & Francis Books

Contents

Illustrations

Figures

Tables

Introduction

From the very beginning of my clinical training, addiction has been the topic that captured my interest more than any other. I vividly recall that, as a young therapist and researcher still in training, my curiosity was not primarily drawn to the substance itself or to its biochemical effects – important as these undoubtedly are. What fascinated me, rather, was everything that lay beneath the surface of addictive behaviour.[1]

Over time, I began to understand that many stories of addiction are held together by an urgent attempt to silence an inner pain devoid of words, form, or regulatory capacity. An unbearable pain that burns, overwhelms, and threatens to engulf the person's entire existence. I came to believe that this was what drove the repeated and compulsive use of drugs.

In those years, I learned that among people who use substances there circulates an expression as crude as it is extraordinarily evocative: "to have the monkey on one's back". This phrase refers to a physical and psychological condition in which the individual experiences the crushing weight of an oppressive force, perceived as more powerful than their own will. For such individuals, substance use – as well as so-called behavioural addictions – while devastating the body and weakening the self, represents the only known strategy for survival. It is a strategy fully embedded within a psychopathological framework, which is why I prefer to use the term addiction[2] rather than pathological dependence or simply dependence. Whereas pathological dependence refers primarily to a physiological condition of need, addiction is better understood as a psychopathological organization grounded in loss of control and, as I will argue in this book, in the structural dissociation of the self. Within this configuration, the addictive-object assumes a dissociative function of self-medication and psychic survival.

At this point, I would like to offer a clarification. Speaking of addiction in pathological terms does not mean – at least for me – reducing it to a medical model that ultimately regards the addicted person as merely ill, nor adopting a nosographic perspective that separates the symptom from the relational and biographical context in which it takes shape. To situate addiction within the domain of psychopathology instead means recognizing the condition of deep

DOI: 10.4324/9781003325314-1

suffering in which the person finds themselves – a condition that cannot be understood if isolated from developmental trajectories, early relational experiences, and the ways in which the self has attempted to organize itself in the face of overwhelming emotional states.

From this perspective, psychopathology is not conceived as a static diagnostic label, but as a clinical and epistemological lens that allows us to interrogate psychic functioning in its complexity. It is in this sense that I propose an integration of the idiographic and nomothetic models: the former indispensable for grasping the irreducible singularity of the individual's history and their specific modes of suffering; the latter necessary for identifying recurring configurations of mental functioning and for developing shareable theoretical frameworks.

Indeed, I believe that knowledge of psychic (or somato-psychic) phenomena cannot be conceived either as the mere description of uniqueness or as the abstraction of general rules valid independently of context, but rather as a dynamic process in which the idiographic and the nomothetic are constantly and creatively intertwined. It is precisely within this fertile tension that addiction can be understood not as a pathology of the object or of behaviour, but as the expression of a psychopathological organization of the self, rooted in unintegrated traumatic experiences and in structural difficulties of affect regulation – or, as Winhall (2021, p. 12) aptly states, "an embodied response to emotional dysregulation".

With regard to the central role of the body and affect in addictive behaviours, there is an experience from those years that has remained deeply etched in my memory and marked a turning point in my understanding of addiction. It was neither a theoretical acquisition nor a simple step in my training, but a clinical encounter that left a lasting imprint on my conception of addictive behaviours and on how I think about the suffering underlying them.

I have also written about this experience in my 2017 book on enactment. At the time, I was a trainee at a public addiction service in Palermo, moving through those spaces with restless curiosity, countless questions, and very few tools to confront the complexity unfolding before me each day. It was then that I encountered a patient who profoundly challenged me – not through language, as we initially exchanged very few words, but through something far more bodily and visceral.

I remember that every time he entered the building, a sharp, acrid smell would permeate the space. It was a foul smell that announced his presence, seeping through the walls, making it difficult to remain in the room, difficult even to breathe or think. His body, emanating that overwhelming smell, seemed to repel any possibility of contact, any opening to relationship. And yet, within that excess, a message was concealed: a silent and desperate request to be seen, to be recognized – in other words, to be helped. That unpleasant odour became a kind of implicit test: a way of testing the other's capacity to remain, not to flee, to tolerate the stench of his pain. The more one defended oneself from the sensory impact of his presence, the higher the wall that rose between him and the world.

Only later did I understand that what he was *enacting* was a *non-symbolized, pre-verbal memory.* At the time, however, I simply felt lost. My supervisor explained to me that this patient had never accepted psychotherapy; he came solely to receive his methadone dose. When he arrived, he would lie down on the chairs in the waiting room – arranged by him in a row – and fall asleep, or remain in a state of torpor while awaiting his turn. Perhaps in order not to feel. Perhaps not to feel himself. Perhaps also not to feel the other, who for him had always been a traumatic, dangerous other to be avoided.

In those years, I had no strategy. No clinical plan. And yet something within me – something I could not have explained at the time – led me to sit beside him. And so I did. In silence. For a few minutes. Without speaking and without expecting anything. It was not a technique, nor a learned intervention; today I would say that I allowed the patient to be together with me in a state of "safe immobility". It was simply what, in that moment, felt right to do. With hindsight, I believe we were engaged in a form of non-verbal communication mediated by our right hemispheres (Schore, 2001) – more specifically, a communication between our non-repressed unconscious minds.

Within the space that emerged between the two of us, something in him began to find a pathway towards expression. I continued in this way for months. Every time I saw him, I sat beside him, without expectations or pressure. Over time, he began to register my presence. He knew I was there, sitting next to him without any demand for change, correction, or judgement. And perhaps precisely for this reason, he did not experience me as a threat.

Then one day, without warning, he broke the silence. He asked to begin meeting in therapy sessions. I accepted immediately. In that moment, I had – for the first time – the sense that I could enter his inner world (his mindset). His narratives – fragmented yet extraordinarily vivid – opened a window onto an ancient and profound pain that had never found anyone willing to listen to. The unpleasant odour that had saturated the service for months began to reveal its deeper meaning. It was the smell of trauma: of early experiences of neglect and violence, of the emotional chaos of his first attachment relationships with frightening parental figures.

That pain was inscribed in his body – in his skin, muscles, breath, and bones. As I have explored in other works (Craparo, 2017; 2026; Caretti & Craparo, 2008; Caretti, Craparo et al., 2005), and as I will elaborate in the chapters that follow, emotional trauma takes root in the body even before it does in the mind. The body retains memory and becomes the primary medium of communication. Thus, through his body, that young man had begun – without knowing it – to ask for help. And what he was seeking was nothing other than a presence willing to take care of that request.

The aim of this book is to explore, from a developmental–relational perspective, the role of trauma and dissociation in the aetiopathogenesis of addictive behaviours. I will refer in particular to the construct of dissociative trauma (Craparo, 2026), considering addictions as trauma-related disorders, alongside conditions such as PTSD, complex PTSD, borderline personality disorder, eating disorders, and psychotic disorders.

With regard to dissociation, a distinction will be drawn between structural dissociation and dissociation understood as an active psychic defence. Although different, both share a fundamental function: to ensure psychological survival. However, whereas structural dissociation derives from overwhelming and disorganizing emotional states, defensive dissociation may be understood as a somato-psychic refuge – associated, in addictions, with the compulsive need to use a addictive-object (alcohol, substances, the internet, sex, food, and so forth) – into which the individual retreats in order to counteract the activation of traumatic memories present in one or more dissociated parts of the personality.

Precisely because the patient's personality is involved, I will refer to the three organizations – neurotic, borderline, and psychotic – as described by Kernberg (1984). A significant finding emerging from both clinical experience and our research is that addicted patients rarely fall within a neurotic organization; rather, they tend to exhibit borderline or psychotic organizations. For this reason, differences will be highlighted between symptomatology rooted in a neurotic structure and that which has its roots in borderline or psychotic structures.

After an in-depth exploration of the psychological and neurobiological mechanisms implicated in addiction – with particular attention to Porges' polyvagal theory (2001, 2011) – the book will focus on trauma- and dissociation-oriented treatments. From this perspective, the importance of a form of therapeutic participation that is not merely technical but deeply human will be emphasized: an active, sensitive, honest, and curious presence, capable of contributing to the co-construction of an embodied setting experienced as a safe and creative space. It is within such a framework that the patient can gradually move from a mode of mere survival towards a fuller and more deeply felt experience of being alive.

In particular, attention will be directed towards an integrated approach that begins with the body and with bottom-up work, privileging clinical interventions that start from how the patient experiences bodily sensations and affective states, and progressively lead towards their conscious understanding. From a neurobiological standpoint, this entails linking information originating in the right hemisphere with left-hemisphere functions, and accomplishing a fundamental shift: from experience to understanding, rather than the reverse. In other words, it involves integrating bottom-up and top-down processes, facilitating a transformation in the very language of experience – from an empty word, devoid of emotional resonance, to a full word capable of containing and conveying a deeper affective, relational, and symbolic understanding.

Notes

1 This term is used to denote addictive behaviour in a broad sense, including traditional substance-related addictions.

2 In Roman law, the *addictus* was an insolvent debtor who, following a public legal act (*addictio*), was assigned to the creditor, thereby losing his personal freedom. Although not formally a slave, he found himself in a condition of subjugation and coercive constraint that deprived him of autonomy and legal identity.

Chapter 1

General Aspects of the Concept of Addiction

Since addictions first became an object of study, what has struck researchers most forcefully is their multifaceted and polyhedral nature. They appear like a prism with many faces: each author, each theory, each clinical orientation seems to grasp an authentic and meaningful aspect of the phenomenon, yet without ever exhausting its complexity. It is as though the field were governed by an epistemological Dodo Bird Verdict: everyone is, in some sense, right, and precisely for this reason no one can claim with absolute certainty to have fully understood the phenomenon. This apparent 'democracy of interpretations' nevertheless reveals, between the lines, the profound frustration of those who investigate this syndrome – the sometimes desolate feeling of having grasped only a small fragment of a much broader clinical enigma.

When I first approached the study of addiction, I formed a conviction that has progressively consolidated over the years: reducing addiction to the mere, almost mechanical repetition of a consumptive behaviour is not only simplistic, but profoundly misleading, as well as harmful both in terms of treatment and in terms of the social perception of the addicted person, who is all too often labelled as weak, licentious, spoiled, or ill.

Moreover, to regard the 'addictive-object' as the ultimate target of addiction is to stop at the surface of the problem – a surface that is frequently deceptive. An exclusive focus at this level has led, for example, some clinicians and researchers to privilege the study of the chemical properties of the substance of abuse and its effects on the organism, losing sight of the social, individual, relational, and developmental dimensions involved. In reaction to this, others have emphasized social or developmental aspects, or intrapsychic processes, while neglecting the biological and chemical components at play.

As Hari (2005) writes,

> We still think of addiction as mainly caused by chemical hooks. There's something in the drug that, after a while, your body starts to crave and need. That's what we think addiction is. But chemical hooks are only a minor part of addiction. The other factors, like isolation and trauma, have been proven to be much bigger indicators. Yet, the drug war

DOI: 10.4324/9781003325314-2

> *increases* the biggest drivers of addiction – isolation and trauma – in order to protect potential users from the more *minor* driver of addiction, the chemical hook.
>
> (p. 271)

A comprehensive perspective is therefore required. Addictions are not monolithic phenomena, but *complex configurations of physical and psychic functioning, rooted in developmental histories marked by relational vulnerabilities, interpersonal trauma, and difficulties in affect regulation.*

They do not merely express a compulsive need directed towards a specific addictive-object; rather, they embody a layered and sometimes invisible form of psychic suffering, which has its roots in the body, in implicit memory, and in the traumatic quality of early attachment relationships.

Over the course of twenty years of clinical and research activity, I have been able to explore at multiple levels the relationship between trauma, dissociation, and addiction. This trajectory has led me to formulate a theoretical and clinical framework that I have conceptualized as the *Dissociative Trauma and Affect Dysregulation–Related Addiction Model*. This model offers a developmental–relational framework for understanding addictions not as pathologies of the object, but as *reenactments* – that is, somatic and emotional reactivations – of unintegrated traumatic experiences. At their core lie physical and psychic mechanisms that I will seek to elucidate through an integrated reading, articulated within a psychodynamic perspective.

Before examining these aspects in greater depth, however, it is appropriate to pause and consider addiction from a descriptive standpoint.

What Is an Addiction?

We can approach this question by first addressing a series of related issues, such as: is the use of a drug in itself an expression of a clinical condition? What distinguishes normal use from pathological use? Does pathological drug use reflect a pre-existing psychic distress? Do so-called behavioural addictions share properties with substance-related addictions?

In this chapter, I will attempt to address these questions, as they represent an indispensable preliminary step for understanding the chapters that follow.

With regard to the first question, the answer – quite intuitively – is no. It is possible to use a substance without necessarily falling into excess or becoming addicted to it.

Whether access to a addictive-object is facilitated or not depends on several factors: its degree of availability, its properties (including chemical ones, in the case of substances and alcohol), social perceptions, and the cultural context in which the behaviour of use is embedded. For example, waking up in the morning and drinking a cup of coffee – who among us would consider this a behaviour of clinical relevance? Or drinking a glass of wine at dinner or during a celebration with friends? Probably no one. The same applies to the internet and digital technologies. Their diffusion and everyday use are now such that it's hard to imagine doing without them, and it would be mistaken to consider it pathological to use them.

These considerations inevitably lead us to the second question: where does the line lie between normal use and pathological or addictive use? Discriminating between a healthy behaviour and an addiction represents a clinical challenge that is far from straightforward. Gabor Maté (2008) offers a pragmatic and incisive criterion when he states that all "addictions cause harm; any habit that does not cause harm is, by definition, not an addiction". In this context, harm does not concern physical or psychological health alone, but also involves family relationships, social life, occupational functioning, and the individual's capacity to maintain an existential balance.

In the DSM-5 (2013), substance use disorder is defined as "a cluster of cognitive, behavioural, and physiological symptoms indicating that the individual continues using the substance despite significant substance-related problems" (APA, 2013, p. 481). Substance-related disorders encompass ten separate classes of drugs; in addition, gambling disorder has been included in the manual because "gambling behaviours activate reward systems similar to those activated by drugs of abuse and produce some behavioural symptoms that appear comparable to those produced by the substance use disorders" (*ibidem*). Other forms of behavioural addiction – such as bigorexia, compulsive shopping, sexual addiction, and internet addiction – have instead been excluded from this diagnostic category, as the manual states that the existing literature is not yet sufficient to define the diagnostic criteria and clinical course that would justify their recognition as mental disorders. This decision, however, appears debatable, given that the available scientific evidence is both substantial and convergent in supporting the addictive nature of these behaviours.

That said, it must be acknowledged that the current edition of the DSM has introduced important diagnostic innovations. First, the previous distinction between abuse and dependence, present in the DSM-IV-TR, has been abandoned and subsumed under a single diagnostic category: substance use disorder. This change reflects an effort to conceptualize problematic use not as a dichotomous condition, but as a dimensional continuum of severity (mild, moderate, severe).

To establish a diagnosis, at least two diagnostic criteria must now be met. Another noteworthy innovation introduced by the manual is the inclusion of the criterion of craving. A limitation, however, lies in the fact that craving is not considered a necessary condition for the diagnosis of addiction, despite extensive clinical and research evidence pointing to its central role in the persistence of addictive behaviour and in the risk of relapse.

Broadening the scope to include behavioural addictions, I conceptualize addiction as a *pathological condition characterized by the distorted use of a substance, an object, or a behaviour; a dysfunctional physical and mental state marked by a sense of irresistibility and by the compulsive need for repetition; an invasive condition in which, as noted, craving is present within the framework of an uncontrollable and irrepressible habit that causes clinically significant distress* (Caretti, Craparo, 2005).

Within this state of enslavement that characterizes the individual's relationship with the addictive-object, craving thus represents the core syndromic condition. Although it is a variable dependent on other factors – as will be illustrated in the course of this book – craving can be recognized in the appetitive urgency and the drive to act, experienced as irreducible even at the expense of the individual's will and despite potential negative consequences.

It is not uncommon for many patients, even after completing a rehabilitation programme – for instance within a therapeutic community – to relapse into the use of one or more substances, sometimes with dramatic outcomes such as overdose. This is an issue that inevitably pervades clinical practice and challenges the very notion of 'recovery' understood as the mere cessation of behaviour.

In this regard, I recall a short film presented by a colleague who worked in a therapeutic community. The video told the story of a man, a former alcohol-addicted patient residing in the facility, who spoke about his relationship with alcohol. His account was intense and authentic, capable of bringing listeners close to the subjective experience of addiction, far beyond diagnostic categories.

At the end of the interview, the journalist asked the protagonist an apparently simple question: "What would you change about your past?" The answer was blunt, almost disarming: "Nothing. I would do everything I did again."

Those words deeply struck the audience. They revealed how, even though the man was no longer using alcohol – because he was living in a 'controlled environment' (DSM-5, p. 491) – craving was still present. Not necessarily in an overt form, but as an internal disposition, as an implicit trace that continued to organize his relationship with the substance.

This example highlights how limiting assessment to the cessation or continuation of substance use behaviour, without considering the persistence of craving, is equivalent to observing only the 'crust' of the phenomenon, while losing sight of the deeper mechanisms underlying compulsive behaviour.

It is precisely from this clinical awareness that, together with other colleagues, I developed the *Addictive Behaviour Questionnaire* (ABQ; Caretti et al., 2016), an instrument designed to capture craving in its articulation with dimensions of obsessiveness, impulsivity, and compulsivity (Table 1.1), thus moving beyond the mere observation of manifest behaviour.[1]

Obsessive thinking focused on the behaviour of use, failure of the will to resist the impulse to act, and compulsive repetition constitute the three defining features of the obsessive–impulsive–compulsive spectrum of craving, which is useful in distinguishing non-problematic use from pathological use.

Table 1.1 The Obsessive–Impulsive–Compulsive Spectrum of Craving

OBSESSIVENESS	IMPULSIVITY	COMPULSIVITY
a) Recurrent thoughts and images concerning addictive experiences or addiction-related ideation (e.g. excessive preoccupation with reliving past addictive experiences or with fantasizing about or planning future addictive experiences); b) Thoughts and images related to addictive behaviour are ego-syntonic and are, at the same time, a source of marked anxiety and distress.	a) Restlessness, anxiety, irritability, or agitation when it is not possible to engage in the addictive behaviour; b) Recurrent failure to resist and regulate addictive desires and impulses to engage in addictive behaviour.	a) Repetitive addictive behaviours that the individual feels compelled to enact, even against their own will and despite possible negative consequences, as a result of recurrent addictive fantasies and impaired impulse control; b) Compulsive addictive behaviours or actions are aimed at avoiding or preventing states of distress or at alleviating a dysphoric mood (e.g. feelings of helplessness, irritability, or inadequacy).

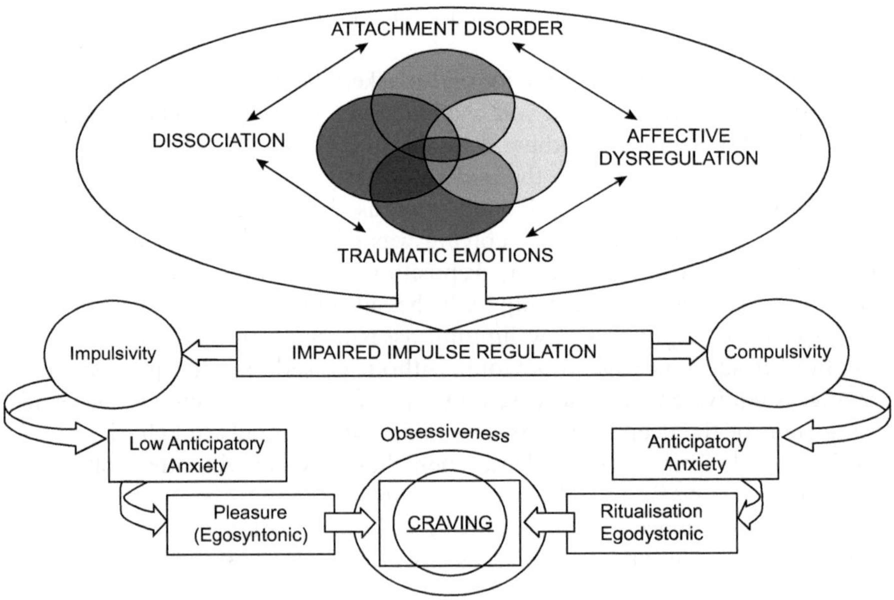

Figure 1.1 Psychodynamic Mechanisms of Craving. Source: Caretti, Craparo, & Schimmenti (2010, p. 117)

In addiction, unlike non-pathological use, this inner drive – difficult to confront and regulate – leads the individual to seek a dissociative somato-psychic refuge, with the aim of attenuating tensions experienced as unbearable, soothing intense and unbearable affective states, compensating for vulnerabilities of the self, and filling psychic voids that are difficult to articulate. Addiction can therefore be understood as a self-reinforcing circular process that organizes behaviour of use around a dissociative core.

Irresistible need, failure of the will, obsessive thoughts, impulsive enactment, and compulsive repetition do not represent isolated phases, but rather interdependent moments of a single defensive movement, within which the addictive-object constitutes the privileged means of regulation.

If addiction is considered as a disorder belonging to the obsessive–impulsive–compulsive spectrum, grounded in dissociative defence mechanisms, it becomes evident that addiction cannot be determined solely by the physiological effects produced by a substance or by a behaviour. Rather, a pre-existing psychopathological condition is present, of which craving represents a natural epiphenomenon.

Together with Vincenzo Caretti and Adriano Schimmenti, I have described the psychodynamic mechanisms underlying craving, which are summarized in the following figure.

As illustrated in the figure, at the core of craving lies a system of traumatic emotions,[2] sustained by psychopathological factors that are rooted in disturbances of the primary attachment relationship. This system gives rise to a deficit in affect regulation capacities and, consequently, to impulse dyscontrol, both at the level of modulation and inhibition. Within this impulsive–compulsive spectrum – which precedes the establishment of the addictive condition – the dysfunctional mental state of craving is further reinforced by multiple orders of bodily sensations, related, as will be discussed shortly, to so-called addiction memories: positive sensations associated with pleasure and relief linked to addiction; negative and painful sensations connected to withdrawal; and, finally, positive sensations related to the regulatory function of addictive behaviour, namely the possibility of counteracting states of physiological hyper- or hypo-arousal through addictive enactment.

These considerations are particularly useful for understanding why approaches to the treatment of addiction based exclusively on re-educational or pharmacological interventions tend to prove ineffective in the long term. The negative consequences of addictive behaviours rarely acquire a transformative value if they are not processed and mentalized by the individual, remaining secondary to the self-regulatory functions that addictive behaviour continues to fulfil and that craving sustains.

This perspective also helps to clarify the frequent comorbidity between addiction and other psychiatric diagnoses. This is not merely a limitation of current diagnostic systems: in most cases, addiction represents the tip of the iceberg of a broader psychopathological condition, the submerged portion of which gradually emerges as the individual's psychic functioning and life experience are explored in greater clinical depth.

Addiction Memory

Neuroimaging studies (Wilson et al., 2004) have shown that exposure to stimuli related to the use of a addictive-object induces marked activation of the amygdala, the anterior cingulate cortex, the orbitofrontal cortex, and the dorsolateral prefrontal cortex. These regions, all involved in emotional regulation, reward evaluation, and executive control, are consistently implicated in craving. It is within this interplay of neural activations that what is referred to as addiction memory is constructed: a deep trace left by the addictive-object in both body and mind, a preferential pathway that the brain tends to follow whenever it recognizes a cue associated with past experiences of use.

This memory is not a passive archive. It is active, selective, and persistent. It is an implicit memory nourished by sensory recollections, bodily perceptions, and emotional states associated with consumption, which it utilizes to orient behaviour. This is why a trigger can suddenly elicit an irresistible urge, linked to the promise of immediate relief, fleeting euphoria, or emotional anaesthesia. Addiction memory may therefore be understood as a somato-psychic memory that integrates the three types of sensations mentioned above: positive sensations evoked by use of the addictive-object; negative sensations associated with the pain of withdrawal; and sensations related to the possibility of counteracting emotional pain through the enactment of addictive behaviour.

This memory becomes part of the individual's very identity, a kind of internal 'programme' that drives the person towards the addictive-object even when conscious will moves in the opposite direction. It is a circuit that repeats itself, a memory that continues to reactivate, sustaining the obsessive–impulsive–compulsive search for the drug: a pull so powerful that it induces the individual to 'lose control', bypassing the cognitive system and evoking an urgency that is difficult to contain.

One might hypothesize that the strengthening of addiction memory is the result of repeated substance use and its effects on the neural circuits involved in reward and motivation systems. While neurochemical mechanisms undoubtedly play a significant role, they alone are insufficient to explain the disruptive force and the tendency towards chronicity that characterize these memories.

Let us imagine a person who uses a substance for the first time. It is highly likely that the experience will be accompanied by pleasant bodily sensations or by a temporary sense of relief. During this phase – often referred to as the 'honeymoon' period – the individual generally experiences intense gratification, accompanied by the feeling of having control over both use and its effects. Any negative consequences are absent, marginal, or actively minimized, thereby sustaining the illusion that the relationship with the drug is manageable, functional, and even beneficial. The body registers this experience, retaining an implicit mnemonic trace linked to pleasure or tension reduction. This bodily memory increases the likelihood of the repetition of the behaviour, functioning as an initial reinforcement.

Over time, however, repeated use tends progressively to shift from the pursuit of pleasure to the need to attenuate painful and dysregulated emotional states. When this occurs, substance use is no longer oriented primarily towards the search for positive sensations, but rather towards the reduction of unbearable affects such as anguish, emptiness, anger, shame, or fear. It is important to emphasize that these affective states are not generated de novo by the substance; rather, they pre-exist and are reactivated by the addictive experience itself.

In this regard, Putnam (1997, pp. 204–5) conceptualizes addiction as:

> the creation of a set of discrete states induced by the substance /and/or behavioural acts associated with use of the substance) – a set that becomes a dominant locus in the larger state space of the individual.
>
> A simplified model of how drug or other addictions develop postulates that the individual creates an initially rewarding altered state of consciousness through the behaviour in question (e.g., smoking crack, playing blackjack, or skydiving). With repeated induction, a set of discrete states with different versions of self, state-dependent memories, behaviours, and regulatory physiology is created. This set of states increasingly comes to dominate the individual's life. In the case of drug use, drug-related states of consciousness act in a competitive, dynamic fashion to displace more conventional states. Often they come to constitute an alternative, often secret life for the individual. We speak of a person as being 'addicted' to a drug when this drug-related set of behavioural states comes to dominate a significant portion of the individual's behaviour.

To understand where addiction memory truly has its roots, it is necessary to shift the focus away from neurobiological processes alone and towards the individual's relational history, particularly experiences of relational trauma and traumatic attachment. As emphasized by Zagaria and colleagues (2024), traumatic attachment is characterized by "varying and long-lasting biological, psychological, and relational consequences resulting from incomplete encoding and integration of emotionally overwhelming experiences within an attachment relationship" (p. 7).

From this perspective, addiction memory may be understood as an embodied and dissociated memory, concerned not merely with the effects of the drug itself, but with the repeated attempt to regulate unmentalized traumatic affects that originate within primary relationships marked by disorganization, unpredictability, or threat. These characteristics render some individuals particularly vulnerable to the repetition of addictive behaviour.

Trauma and Attachment

A substantial body of research (see, for example, the collection edited by Wiechelt & Straussner, 2016) indicates that the vulnerabilities predisposing individuals to the development of addictive behaviours have their roots in developmental deficits in the organization of the self. Such deficits are frequently associated with neglectful or abusive family environments, or with contexts marked by pronounced relational disorganization, in which addictive behaviours among other family members are also commonly observed (Dube et al., 2002; Felitti et al., 1998). These emotional deficits significantly impair the individual's capacity to regulate intense and negative emotional states, to maintain a coherent and realistic sense of self, and to form stable affective relationships.

For example, a review of twelve studies (Leza et al., 2021) showed that Adverse Childhood Experiences[3] (ACEs) were significantly more prevalent among individuals with substance use disorders than in the general population. A large-scale analysis involving over 14,000 European adolescents and young adults (Hughes et al., 2019) found that those who had experienced four or more ACEs were four times more likely to develop problems related to alcohol or drug misuse. Similar findings have also emerged with respect to other forms of addiction, including gambling disorder (Sharma & Sacco, 2015), internet addiction (Hao, Li, Liang, & Geng, 2024), and sexual addiction (Kotera & Rhodes, 2019).

From a developmental–relational perspective, Adverse Childhood Experiences share not only their intrinsically stressful nature, but above all the fact that they occur during sensitive phases of development, directly involve attachment figures, and interfere with fundamental processes of self-development. Such experiences compromise affect regulation capacities, hinder the development of mentalization,[4] and promote the activation of processes of structural dissociation.

Their clinical relevance lies not merely in the events themselves, but rather in the absence of a regulatory, protective, and reparative response from the caregiving environment, which leaves the child alone in the face of overwhelming and non-integrable emotional states. The research cited above suggests that a common logic of functioning recurs across different types of addiction: the addictive-object – whether a substance, the internet, gambling, sex, or other behaviours – is progressively invested as a privileged device for affect regulation and psychic survival.

Notes

1 The questionnaire also allows for the diagnosis of the presence of one of the following four categories of addiction: substance-related addiction, alcohol addiction, gambling addiction, and internet addiction. In addition, a specific section (7DAS) was included, comprising the following seven domains (Caretti, Gori, Craparo et al., 2016), which are frequently associated with addiction:

1. ***Separation anxiety***, for the assessment of difficulties in safely establishing and/or experiencing attachment relationships (insecure attachment);
2. ***Affect dysregulation***, for the assessment of difficulties in identifying, differentiating, modulating, and communicating emotions;
3. ***Somatoform and psychological dissociation***, for the assessment of symptoms related to altered states of consciousness and feelings of estrangement from oneself, one's own body, and others;
4. ***Childhood traumatic experiences***, for the assessment of traumatized mental states associated with experiences of emotional neglect or abuse during childhood;
5. ***Impulse dyscontrol***, for the assessment of difficulties in resisting impulses, compelling urges, or behaviours despite the potential negative consequences of one's actions;
6. ***Compulsive behaviour and ritualization***, for the assessment of the tendency to engage compulsively in repetitive and ritualized behaviours, even when they are harmful to one's health or well-being;
7. ***Obsessive thoughts***, for the assessment of obsessional, recurrent, persistent, and repetitive thinking, as well as difficulties in decision-making.

2 Traumatic emotions (Craparo, 2017) are characterized by a specific nature that distinguishes them from ordinary emotions. First, they are *pre-verbal*, as they lack a psychic representation capable of conferring meaning and rendering them amenable to mentalization. They exhibit a marked *physiological–motor component*: in the absence of reflective processes, their activation translates into sudden, stereotyped, and rigid responses, often experienced by the individual as scarcely controllable. These emotions are also profoundly painful, as the failure of affect identification and modulation processes leads to an amplification of subjective intensity, sustained by a state of pronounced autonomic hyperarousal. Finally, traumatic emotions are *disorganizing*, in that they trigger and maintain processes of *structural dissociation* between different self-states, functioning as a defensive response to conditions of stress experienced by the individual as threatening to psychic survival.

3 Adverse Childhood Experiences (ACEs) encompass a range of traumatic events occurring during childhood and adolescence, and have been shown to exert a significant and enduring impact on the individual's psychological, emotional, relational, and somatic development. In the classical ACE Study model (Felitti et al., 1998), traumatic experiences are organized into three broad domains: abuse (emotional, sexual, and physical), neglect (emotional and physical), and household dysfunction (including domestic violence, substance misuse within the family, caregiver mental illness, parental separation or divorce, and the incarceration of a family member).

4 Mentalization is a process that is:

a) *emotional and embodied*, insofar as it does not consist merely in formulating thoughts about feelings, but also – and above all – in feeling emotions at the very moment they are experienced;
b) *intentional and conscious*, in that feelings and thoughts are always about something, whether belonging to the internal or external world, towards which the individual maintains a receptive and mindful attention;
c) *intersubjective*, as it cannot be separated from an interactional reference involving the sharing and exploration of mental states, which constitutes a conditio sine qua non for the individual's capacity to hold in mind both their own mind and the mind of the other.

Chapter 2

A Developmental–Relational Interpretation of Addiction

The approach I use to understand addiction is developmental–relational in nature. It is therefore appropriate to clarify what I mean by this construct, starting with the term developmental, understood in its dual sense: 1. as a sequence of interconnected 'moments' within individual development; 2. as an evolutionary process in the broader sense.

Both meanings are examined through a psychodynamic lens (Craparo, 2013; 2024). It is important to clarify that I do not use the term 'developmental' as a synonym for progress. Were this the case, we would be inclined to conceive psychopathology as a mere deviation from a supposedly correct or normative pathway, thereby risking a slide into an orthodox and scientistic view historically associated with well-known ideological drifts. For this reason, addiction cannot be interpreted as the outcome of a simple interruption of a developmental process structured around predetermined stages, even though it is undeniable that human development unfolds through phases, each characterized by the acquisition of specific adaptive competences. Rather, the distinctive features of each phase should be understood as expressions of a complex interplay of phenomena that mutually interact, some of which are not necessarily predictable.

In this regard, the concept of *evolutionary contingency* developed within neo-Darwinian theory (Pievani, 2017) proves particularly useful: evolutionary processes are not the product of rigid laws nor of pure chance, but of a concatenation of events whose effects can only be fully understood retrospectively. This does not preclude the possibility of formulating developmental predictions, provided that they are embedded within probabilistic reasoning.

Development cannot be conceived as an engineering or mechanical process, whereby the sum of A, B, and C inevitably leads to outcome Z; nor does it make sense to search for a single 'missing link' capable of explaining, on its own, a complex phenomenon such as addiction. Scientific evidence does not support such an approach. Outcomes may be multiple, and although a certain regularity may sometimes lead to Z, this occurs within a plurality of possible trajectories influenced by personal, biological, and cultural factors that intertwine over time in often unpredictable ways.

DOI: 10.4324/9781003325314-3

With regard to the term 'relational', it is now well established that each individual constructs and organizes their psychic and bodily life through the multiple ways in which they relate to others, beginning – most crucially – in the earliest years of life. Early relationships do not merely constitute the context of development, but represent one of its fundamental matrices. Neuroscientific research (see Schore, 2015; Gallese, 2014) has shown that the quality of caregiving experiences in early life exerts a significant impact on the child's psychological and neurobiological development, profoundly influencing how the child will learn to perceive, regulate, and attribute meaning to their internal states.

From this perspective, the relational dimension draws on the converging contributions of attachment theory, psychoanalysis, and interpersonal neurobiology. It may be stated – not merely metaphorically – that each of us is made of the same substance as the relationships we have lived and internalized. The quality of these relationships shapes the way we perceive the world, experience emotions, think about experience, and act in relation to ourselves and to the environment.

It follows that psychological development cannot be understood as an exclusively intrapsychic process, but rather as the dynamic and ongoing outcome of the encounter between mind, body, and relationship.

The Effects of Traumatic Attachment on Affect Regulation

Having clarified, albeit briefly, what I mean by a developmental–relational perspective, we may now turn to attachment research, which has shown that neglectful or disorganizing primary relationships leave a 'void' not so much in declarative memory as in implicit memory – a domain of mind and body in which certain emotional experiences, although intensely registered at a physiological level, fail to be transformed into shareable and thinkable representations within a secure relational context (Bowlby, 1979; 1980; 1988). In such cases, emotion fails to find an intersubjective container capable of giving it form and remains as bodily activation without symbolization.

At this point, it is useful to distinguish between emotion and feeling. Emotion is first and foremost a neurophysiological and somatic event associated with primary consciousness; feeling, by contrast, implies the capacity to construct an 'idea of the body' when it is perturbed by physiological activation, thereby transforming emotion into an ideational–affective representation that can subsequently be integrated into interpersonal narrative (Taylor, Bagby, & Parker, 1997). When this transformation does not occur, emotional experience remains without mental form: it cannot be thought, named, or located in time. It is in this sense that, within the context of traumatic attachment, certain emotions acquire a specifically traumatizing quality.

I define these experiences as traumatic emotions, since within abusive or neglectful primary relationships they are not processed but remain isolated, unintegrated, and potentially destabilizing for the development of the self. Traumatic emotion becomes clinically visible when stressful events reactivate this unmentalized affective core, renewing emotional confusion and a fragmentation of the self: pain cannot be traversed through a normal elaborative process but tends instead to become fixed, because what should become psychic experience remains an excess of somatic–affective activation.

In the face of stress and the reactivation of traumatic emotions, the individual may resort to substances or behaviours in order to induce alternative somato-sensory states capable of counteracting internal disorganization and the sense of disintegration.

Within this framework, addiction may be understood as a dissociative response. Here, the construct of dissociation does not refer solely to the so-called 'classical' dissociative syndromes, but rather to structural and/or defensive processes that separate unbearable and non-mentalized affective states from conscious experience. Dissociation operates as a disconnection between representations, affects, memories, and self-states, making psychic survival possible in the face of experiences incompatible with the continuity of the self. When such states remain chronically unintegrated, however, the addictive-object becomes invested as an external regulator of what cannot be regulated internally.

What follows is a recursive model: difficulties in affect regulation, traumatic emotions, and dissociative processes mutually reinforce one another, obstructing the possibility of 'learning from experience' (Bion, 1962) and of transforming pain into psychic texture. From this perspective, the addictive-object is not the ultimate aim, but the means through which the individual attempts to anaesthetize or modulate the emergence of unintegrated self-states that retain an implicit memory of non-symbolized and non-integrated – or only partially integrated – experiences. This feature defines what are commonly referred to as traumatic memories, whose core consists of traumatic emotions that tend to be re-enacted in the form of re-enactment when the individual comes into contact with specific environmental or relational triggers.

The result is that the person remains anchored to a traumatic past from which they struggle to emancipate themselves, repeatedly reproducing affective, bodily, and behavioural patterns that continue to exert a powerful influence on present life. This condition, widely confirmed in clinical practice, demonstrates that addictions – whether to alcohol, substances, the internet, gambling, or anything else – cannot be adequately understood without taking into account the persistence and disorganizing force of relational wounds that have left a lasting imprint on the self.

In Figure 2.1, I represent the addictive process as a circular one. Within this process, addiction memories are rooted in traumatic memories located within a dissociated part of the personality. Addiction memories, in turn, fuel craving, which translates into repetitive behaviours capable of inducing a somato-psychic state of dissociative withdrawal, used as a refuge to anaesthetize overwhelming tensions.[1]

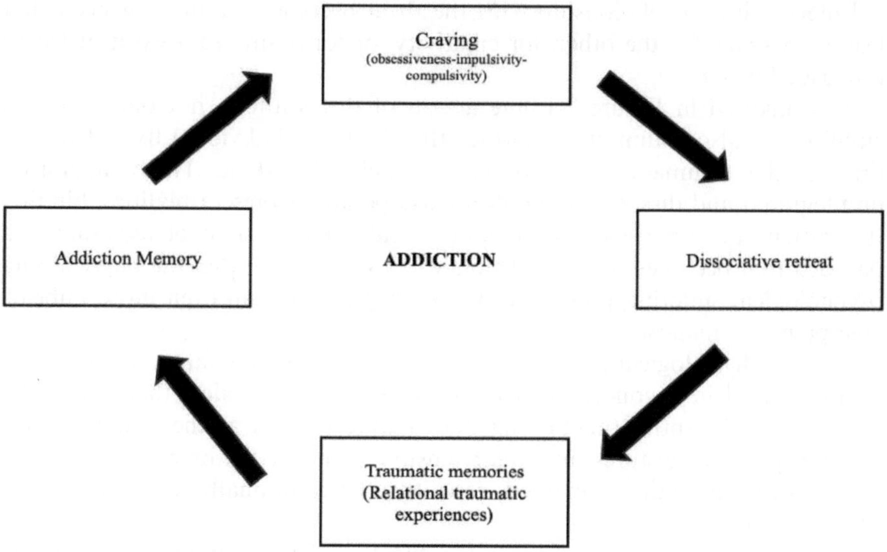

Figure 2.1 The Circular Process of Addiction

In light of the role that trauma plays in addiction, I believe that clinicians should have a solid training in psychotraumatology. Indeed, the understanding of addiction cannot be separated from situating it within the complex network of interpersonal traumas that, in the majority of cases, constitute its generative core. In other words, it is not possible to fully grasp the nature of addiction without recognizing the crucial role of trauma and relational wounds that profoundly shape the individual's emotional, bodily, and interpersonal functioning.

These wounds imprint terrifying sensations on the person's intimate experience, sensations that hinder the development of a sense of personal vitality, internal safety, and genuine curiosity towards the world. As Gabor Maté (2018), psychotraumatologist and leading expert in the treatment of addiction, author of the well-known *In the Realm of Hungry Ghosts*, observes, every addictive behaviour represents an attempt to resolve "the problem of emotional pain, of overwhelming stress, of lost connection, of loss of control, of a deep discomfort with the self". It follows that, as Maté suggests, the clinically relevant question is not so much "*Why the addiction*?" as "*Why the pain*?" (*ibidem*).

The addicted patient seeks relief from internal states of insecurity and unbearable affects. Addiction thus becomes a desperate attempt to bring emotions and sensations that would otherwise be overwhelming back within a tolerable threshold – within what Siegel has defined the window of tolerance, which in traumatized/addicted patients is narrower than in non-traumatized individuals.

Entering into a relationship with the drug becomes a totalizing need that leaves no space for the other, for creativity, or for desire. In a word, it leaves no space for life.

As suggested in Figure 2.1, the action of drugs affects not only pleasure circuits, but also traumatic memories that keep the individual fixated on the time of the trauma and the malaise associated with it. These memories, unintegrated and dissociated, continue to operate as present realities, binding the patient to a persistent and paradoxical internal state of *suffering* – a paradox that becomes comprehensible when we consider that the physical and psychological suffering produced by the drug replaces an even more unbearable pain and malaise.[2]

From a physiological standpoint, the activation of traumatic memories can be recognized in a condition of continuous autonomic alert that permeates the individual's entire functioning and manifests both at the bodily level – through posture, gestures, muscular tension – and at the expressive and linguistic level, through fragmented, repetitive, or emotionally urgent modes of communication.

In this context, substance use takes the form of an attempt to modulate extreme neurovegetative states, intervening where affective and symbolic regulation is compromised. It is as if the body were catapulted into the past, reacting to stimuli perceived as threatening and activating automatic defensive responses. As Van der Kolk (2014) states, the traumatized person is "more there than here", more in the past than in the present. The activation of traumatic memories entails a loosening of the *function of reality*, accompanied by a reduction in the capacities for *presentification* and *personification* (Janet, 1909). The former manifests as difficulty remaining connected to the present moment; the latter is expressed as a sense of estrangement from oneself, due to dissociated parts that may partially or totally take control of consciousness. This experience is clearly recognizable in patients' words, such as: "I wasn't in control of myself", "I wanted to stop, but I couldn't", "It wasn't me at that moment".

One of my patients addicted to crack – G. – had given a name, Bronson, to the dissociated part of his personality that he experienced as responsible for his addictive behaviours: "Bronson is angry, vengeful; he wants nothing but to get high and then get high again, without thinking about the consequences. The real problem is that when he shows up, I completely lose control. He's my *monkey on my back.*" In his spontaneous language, the presence of a dissociated configuration of bodily and mental states clearly emerged, taking over in moments of heightened vulnerability and dragging him towards compulsive drug use. For him, Bronson was not a metaphor, but a real internal presence, experienced as alien, intrusive, and uncontrollable.

This description vividly conveys what many patients experience: addiction as a dissociated internal force, organized around urgent needs for escape, anaesthesia, and self-medication, rooted in the reactivation of unintegrated traumatic memories.

Stephen Porges' polyvagal theory (2011) allows for a further deepening of this process from a neurobiological perspective. According to Porges, addiction can be understood as a maladaptive strategy activated through sympathetic mobilization or dorsal-vagal numbing in response to stimuli 'neurocepted' as threatening. The reactivation of traumatic memories thus facilitates dissociative enactments: fight-or-flight responses (sympathetic system), or states of collapse and emotional shutdown (dorsal-vagal system), both of which are supported and reinforced by the use of the addictive-object. Porges (2022) writes:

> Addiction, from a polyvagal perspective, reflects an unsuccessful strategy to reduce the impact of threat by numbing or mobilizing. Addiction can appear to successfully mask, distort, or numb feelings of threat. Interestingly, the strategy of numbing and masking seems to follow implicit strategies frequently employed to foster a dissociation between feelings and actions, and frequent valiant attempts to prevent bodily feelings from disrupting intentional behaviours. However, unlike the neurobiological potency of sociality in generating feelings of safety, these strategies fail, and over time exacerbate feelings of threat.
>
> A polyvagal perspective of addiction focuses on the attempted use of addictive substances or behaviours to damp underlying feelings of threat. This perspective frames the client's behaviour within a quest to feel safe. Unfortunately, feeling safe is dependent on an autonomic state that can only efficiently be reached through sociality, while recruiting ancient neurobiologically based survival strategies that are insensitive to the intentions of higher brain circuits will fail
>
> (p. 16).

The author highlights how addictive behaviours further weaken integrative capacities and social connection, trapping the person in dysfunctional survival strategies. For this reason, similarly to what occurs in traumatized patients – for example those diagnosed with post-traumatic stress disorder – patients with addiction diagnoses can also be considered survivors, who resort to extreme strategies to cope with an environment experienced as hostile and poorly regulating. The cost of this repeated recourse, however, is extremely high, as it leads to a progressive loss of the capacity to live adaptively and in connection with the surrounding world.

If this is the case – if addiction configures itself as a survival attempt, albeit dysfunctional, in response to the present-day reactivation of dissociative traumatic memories – then the question that naturally arises is: why not consider addiction as a specific trauma-related disorder?

Indeed, this is how I conceptualize it: a trauma-related disorder, although, as I will discuss in Chapter Three, I prefer to speak of dissociative trauma.

Let us return to G. He is the second-born child in a family of four: mother, father, older brother, and himself. The father, a silent and withdrawn man, had been abandoned in a convent at birth and had never known his parents. The mother is described as emotionally unstable, harsh, and often violent. G. recalls numerous episodes in which he was brutally beaten by his mother, sometimes for trivial reasons, without any intervention from the father. Although the father had almost never physically abused the children – except on one occasion, at the insistence of his wife – he was unable to offer any gestures of tenderness or protection.

The maternal family history was marked by severe economic hardship, emotional neglect, and abuse: G.'s mother had grown up with two alcoholic, violent, and emotionally absent parents. Her sister had also lived a life marked by distress, with repeated incarcerations for drug dealing and prostitution. In this climate, both G. and his brother, three years older, developed rebellious and oppositional behaviours from early childhood. "My brother and I were wild kids, avoided by others. As teenagers we started heavy use of heroin, cannabis, alcohol, and then crack," G. recounts.

The pain G. carries is profound and unbearable – a pain he attempts to anaesthetize through substance use: heroin and cannabis in adolescence, alcohol and later crack in adulthood. As Gabor Maté (2008) notes, drugs can become an emotional anaesthetic, an antidote to terrifying emptiness, a tonic against fatigue, boredom, alienation, and inadequacy, an anti-stress agent and a lubricant for existence. In G.'s case, it is the implicit memory of intergenerational trauma that shapes his reactions: events that have torn the psychic fabric and hindered his emotional and social development.

During a session, G. reports having just returned from a visit to his parents: "We had one of our usual fights. But all in all, it went fine. I'm fine." Shortly afterwards, almost casually, he adds: "It's mathematical – every time I go back to my parents' place, I get the flu."

I ask him what bodily sensations he is experiencing at that moment. "I struggle to breathe. I feel rigid. I have difficulty speaking." The bodily rigidity evoked the same freezing state he had experienced as a child during maternal assaults. In that 'flu', experienced as a chilled and contracted body, a memory of terror seems to resonate: a dissociated part of the self that retains the traces of trauma and activates ancient autonomic survival responses, particularly freezing. It is as if G. were saying with his body: "It's mathematical – every time I go back to my parents, I freeze with terror."

He also recounts a dream he had after returning from the visit. He is in his childhood home. His mother, wielding a wooden club, smashes walls, chairs, doors, until she destroys the only escape route. G. tries to speak but cannot: his mouth is full of pieces of glass that cut him every time he moves it. He wakes up agitated and distressed. Even in recounting it, he is visibly activated. The dream represents a clear re-enactment of his traumatic memories: entrapment, terror, inability to communicate, helplessness in the face of maternal violence.

The dreams of patients with addiction are often striking in their concrete intensity, crudity, and aggressiveness. G.'s dream is an emblematic example: a scene that re-presents, in an extremely realistic form, the traumatic world – external and internal – from which he has tried to escape for years, first through rebellion, then through substances. Yet that impulse, which initially functioned as a survival strategy, ultimately traps G., sabotaging every attempt to approach new and healthier ways of living and feeling safe. When the saboteur (Bronson) appears, G. experiences it as an invitation to use the substance: "Forget it, what are you waiting for?" Sometimes it is a seductive voice, at other times aggressive, violent, angry. Born to protect the individual from an unsafe environment, it gradually rigidifies into an internal presence that limits him and rejects any change as if it were a threat.

This is why addictive behaviours sometimes appear to take on a masochistic quality: the search for a more tolerable suffering as an alternative to something terrifying.

For Fairbairn (1952; 1963), when a child is exposed to rejecting relational experiences, they tend to introject the rejecting parent as a bad internal object. This introjection serves a fundamental defensive function, as it preserves the illusion of the existence of a good external object. The internal saboteur is the result of this internalization of the bad object – an extreme solution aimed at avoiding the loss of a bond that would be experienced as unbearable. As Vittorio Lingiardi (2025) states, the internal saboteur "is the part of us that has remained loyal to the rejecting or abusive object in order not to lose the bond: a voice from the past that speaks in the present [...]. When we are neglected, maltreated, or abused by those who should care for us, Fairbairn argues, the mind, in order to protect itself, divides experience into internal objects: gratifying, exciting, and rejecting. [...] The internal saboteur is the product of an identification with the rejecting parental figure, idealized as loving but subsequently introjected as absent, destructive, and judgemental. It is the part of the ego that embodies the hiss of devaluation, the ferocity of criticism, and the humiliation of punishment" (pp. 101–102, my translation).

In the context of addiction, the internal saboteur represents a dissociated part of the self that, while enacting survival strategies, ultimately obstructs any attempt at change. It constitutes the legacy of a traumatic attachment identification[3] with deeply dysfunctional neglectful figures and makes use of compulsive drug consumption as an immediately available means to regulate, sedate, or anaesthetize a profound and intimate malaise.

What originally had a protective function – albeit dysfunctional for psychological and physical health – gradually transforms into a mechanism that undermines self-trust, reactivates traumatic schemas, and keeps the individual trapped in rigid and maladaptive coping modes. As Jan Winhall (2021) observes: "Addiction is something that helps you in the short term, harms you in the long term, and you can't get free from it" (p. 1).

In sum, the internal saboteur is the expression of autonomic survival states (fight, flight, freeze, or collapse) that continue to organize the individual's experience long after the original traumatic context has passed.

The Construct of the Addictive-Object

I have used the expression addictive-object to refer not only to a category that includes both psychotropic substances and addictive behaviours in which no substance is ingested (such as sex, food, gambling, the internet, and so forth), but above all in a psychoanalytic sense.

In Freudian theory, the object is the correlate of the drive, and more specifically that which allows the attainment of its aim, namely satisfaction. It may be a person – for example, the mother – a partial object, such as the breast, or a phantasmatic object; in every case, however, the object is inseparable from the bodily experience of the gratification or frustration of the drive.

Post-Freudian theorization – by Klein, Bion, Winnicott, and the entire object relations tradition – has profoundly complexified this notion, articulating the internal, symbolic, and transformative nature of the object. I do not intend here to engage with the vast psychoanalytic literature concerning the different theoretical interpretations of the object; rather, I wish to outline some specific features of the addictive-object as they emerge from clinical experience.

A first salient feature is its radically concrete nature. The addictive-object has no symbolic function: it does not refer to something else, nor does it represent anything that has been repressed within the dynamic unconscious. It is not supported by a representational apparatus and cannot be described as a transitional object, insofar as it does not symbolically mediate between inner and outer worlds, nor does it open a space for meaning-making. Instead, it evokes only bodily or affective sensations (linked to the non-repressed unconscious), such as the euphoric activation induced by cocaine or the opioid release associated with morphine. The bond with the addictive-object is therefore immediate and mediated exclusively by the sensations it elicits.

For these reasons, the addictive-object bears closer resemblance to what Bollas (2019) has conceptualized an "alternative object". The alternative object emerges when the transitional space fails: it does not function as a bridge towards reality but replaces it; it gives form to an "other" internal world, a somato-psychic retreat in which survival is possible through withdrawal from the pain of contact with the other. Bollas describes it as a "playless" space, ritualized in nature, a place in which to deposit "dead selves", a kind of psychic cemetery inhabited by spectral objects.[4]

The somato-psychic space organized around the addictive-object is not generative of symbols or thought, but rather a domain of immediate regulation, in which the object is used as an instrument to modulate states of physiological hyper- or hypo-arousal. In this sense, it is not a transformative object but a sedative one: it does not facilitate the working-through of affect, but anaesthetizes it; it does not open a space for thought, but suspends it. It enables survival at the cost of the possibility of feeling alive.

Notes

1 Trauma is not inscribed solely in narrative memory or in conscious psychic life but leaves deep and enduring traces in the body. It is the body, even before the mind, that is traumatized.
2 Distinguishing it from disturbance, René Kaës (2012) defines malaise as that which causes the very foundations of psychic life and its cultural correlates to waver: malaise calls into question the capacity to be and to exist (p. 307).
3 By Traumatic Attachment Identification I refer to a process through which the self unconsciously organizes around an internalized traumatic attachment, in response to early conditions of relational threat, supported by dissociation and oriented towards the preservation of the bond rather than the integration of experience.
4 In psychoanalysis, phantasy refers to unconsciously symbolized contents related to repressed desire, which is why it tends to *torment* the individual. The spectre, by contrast, concerns non-represented and pre-symbolic contents. It is associated with internal objects deprived of vitality and endowed with a primitive aggressiveness which, rather than tormenting, *terrorize.*

Chapter 3

The Neurobiology of Addiction

Over the past few decades, neuroscientific research has radically transformed our understanding of addiction. What was once attributed to moral weakness or a lack of willpower is now recognized as a complex condition rooted in profound alterations of brain systems that regulate motivation, emotion, learning, memory, and behavioural control. This perspective does not eliminate the subjective and relational dimensions of addiction; rather, it integrates them by demonstrating how the neural circuits involved can account for the compulsive force of addictive behaviour, vulnerability to relapse, and the difficulty of discontinuing a pattern of use that the individual knows to be harmful.

Koob and Volkow (2016) have conceptualized addiction as a recurrent cycle articulated in three phases: binge/intoxication, withdrawal/negative affect, and preoccupation/anticipation. These phases are not isolated compartments, but moments within a progressive process in which the same brain circuits are repeatedly engaged and cumulatively modified. In the early stages, impulsivity predominates: the immediate desire for pleasure or relief drives substance use. Over time, however, motivation shifts, and use is no longer oriented towards pleasure, but towards avoiding the distress associated with withdrawal. It is precisely in this transition from positive reinforcement to negative reinforcement that compulsivity and behavioural rigidity become entrenched – a formulation consistent with the obsessive–impulsive–compulsive spectrum discussed in the first chapter.

The three phases of the cycle correspond to a progressive dysregulation of three fundamental brain systems. The basal ganglia, involved in reward processing and habit formation, are initially 'hijacked' by the drug, which produces a rapid increase in dopamine release in the nucleus accumbens. With repeated use, however, dopamine release becomes less associated with the drug itself and more with the stimuli that predict – places, people, objects, and emotional states. These cues acquire incentive salience and become capable of eliciting craving and drug-seeking behaviour even in the absence of the substance. Behavioural control gradually shifts towards dorsal striatal circuits, which are more rigid and automatized. Drug-seeking thus progressively becomes a highly automatized habit, increasingly resistant to voluntary modulation.

DOI: 10.4324/9781003325314-4

When the substance is unavailable, the individual enters the withdrawal or negative affect phase, dominated by a profound dysregulation of stress systems. Reward neurochemistry falls below baseline levels, generating a pervasive sense of emptiness, a loss of motivation, and an inability to derive pleasure from ordinary activities. In this vulnerable context, stress-related systems such as corticotropin-releasing factor (CRF), noradrenaline, and dynorphin become activated, producing irritability, agitation, anxiety, and dysphoria. Koob and Volkow describe this condition as an allostatic state: a pathological new equilibrium in which the brain 'expects' the presence of the substance in order to function within a tolerable range. Substance use resumes not to obtain pleasure, but to alleviate escalating emotional and physiological pain.

In the third phase – preoccupation and anticipation – craving becomes prominent and a significant impairment of executive functions emerges. The prefrontal cortex, responsible for impulse control, the evaluation of consequences, and emotional regulation, shows reduced functional capacity, resulting in diminished inhibitory control, poorly considered decision-making, and a heightened vulnerability to stress. The insula, which plays a crucial role in interoceptive awareness, amplifies the subjective experience of need, making it difficult to distinguish between genuine physiological requirements and learned impulses. Desire is thus experienced as something that 'happens by itself', often in direct opposition to conscious intentions.

The model proposed by these authors conceptualizes addiction as a spiralling cycle of dysregulation involving reward and anti-reward brain mechanisms, progressively intensifying and leading to compulsive substance use. Counter-adaptive processes – such as opponent processes that normally serve to restore homeostatic balance in reward functioning – fail to return to the normal homeostatic range, resulting instead in an allostatic condition. These counter-adaptive processes are thought to be mediated by two mechanisms: within-system neuroadaptations and between-system neuroadaptations (Koob & Bloom, 1988). Within-system neuroadaptation refers to cellular or molecular changes within a given reward circuit that initially support the heightened reward-processing associated with addiction but ultimately result in a reduction of overall reward function.

I suggest that this neurocircuitry framework can be fruitfully integrated with Stephen Porges' Polyvagal Theory, which elucidates how behavioural responses – including addictive behaviours – derive from the continuous modulation of the autonomic nervous system (ANS) in the service of safety. From Porges' perspective, many addictive behaviours are not merely the consequence of an altered reward circuit but adaptive responses of an organism unable to access states of calm and social connection. When neuroception – the automatic and implicit system that detects cues of safety or threat – is chronically oriented towards defence, as often occurs in traumatized and addicted individuals, social engagement becomes difficult or inaccessible. Addiction then emerges as a (dysfunctional) substitute for physiological regulation, offering temporary relief while simultaneously trapping the organism in states of hyperarousal or collapse.

Building on this framework, Jan Winhall (2021) integrated polyvagal theory with Gendlin's somatic practices, developing the Felt Sense Polyvagal Model, which places the body at the centre of knowledge and regulation. Through access to the felt sense, patients learn to recognize their autonomic states, detect subtle bodily signals that precede loss of control, and identify transitions between sympathetic mobilization, dorsal vagal collapse, and ventral vagal connection. Addictive behaviours appear as attempts to move rapidly from a painful state towards a minimal equilibrium, albeit one that is often transient and harmful – in other words, addiction substitutes for ventral vagal connection.

Another neurobiological hypothesis that I have found particularly useful for understanding addiction, and which integrates well with the perspectives discussed above, concerns 'thalamic deafferentation', a concept that highlights an additional aspect of the somato-psychic mechanisms of addiction, namely structural dissociation. Specifically, Lanius, Paulsen, and Corrigan (2014) hypothesize that the core of structural dissociation and the development of separate self-states are due to the deafferentation of basic affective circuits induced by endogenous opioids released under threat. These opioids inhibit thalamic functioning, leading to a separation of affective states from ordinary conscious awareness. In other words, when the body is exposed to pain or threat, it automatically releases endogenous opioids that inhibit thalamic transmission, thereby reducing cortical access to subcortical signals and diminishing the conscious perception of pain. A common everyday example is the experience of falling and not immediately feeling pain, which emerges only several minutes later – an instance of thalamic deafferentation.

According to Lanius and colleagues (2014), the repeated experience of painful events that induce recurrent deafferentation may lead to a transition from peritraumatic dissociation to structural dissociation.

These three models should not be understood as competing alternatives, but as complementary frameworks. The first precisely describes the alternation of reward, stress, and executive control circuits throughout the course of addiction; the second explains why these alterations take hold more readily in nervous systems shaped by trauma and deprived of secure interpersonal regulation; the third elucidates the neurobiological basis of addiction as a dissociative response to emotional pain. Addictive compulsivity thus derives not only from changes in dopaminergic receptors or transcription factors, but also from the body's difficulty in orienting towards connection. The allostasis described by Koob can be understood in relation to an autonomic nervous system that is unable to settle; incentive salience can be viewed as a distorted attempt to regulate overwhelming states of activation; executive dysfunction reflects the loss of reflective capacity when the ANS is trapped in defensive states (fight, flight, freeze, collapse). Thalamic deafferentation further links addictive behaviours to the need to retreat into neurobiological states of detachment in order not to feel pain, contributing – through repetition – to the consolidation of dissociative organization.

All these features characterize both substance-related addictions and so-called behavioural addictions. As Lewis (2015) notes, “the neural consequences of behavioural addictions indicate the same cellular consequences and the same biological alterations underlying substance addiction” (p. 23).

The clinical implication of neurobiological research is that the treatment of addicted patients cannot be limited to simply ‘removing the drug’, but must provide new forms of regulation, new experiences of interpersonal connection, and new possibilities for neurophysiological reorganization, alongside a transformation of the psychic world.

Chapter 4

Need or Desire?

Precisely because the addictive-object evokes sensations that function as a dissociative refuge against an unthinkable – and therefore unbearable – pain, its use does not arise from desire but from need, that is, from craving.

In psychoanalysis, the distinction between desire and need represents a fundamental theoretical point. Desire, governed by the pleasure principle (Freud, 1900; 1920), can emerge only in the presence of a sufficiently regulated body–mind, capable of tolerating absence and of representing what is not yet present. Desire introduces distance, opens a space for symbolization, and allows for the postponement of satisfaction.

Among the authors who have most deeply explored the concept of desire, Lacan (1958–1959/2021) stands out for having highlighted its structural coincidence with lack, arguing that desire can never be fully satisfied by a real object. The object of desire – *objet petit a* in Lacanian terminology – is not something that can be attained or possessed, but rather that which causes desire. It is the object that sets desire in motion; for this reason, Lacan defines it as the cause of desire rather than an object of satisfaction. In *The Language of Psychoanalysis*, Laplanche and Pontalis (2018) state:

> This perspective has led Lacan to distinguish desire from concepts with which it is often confused, such as need and demand. Need is directed towards a specific object and is satisfied by it. Demands are formulated and addressed to others; where they are still aimed at an object, this is not essential to them, since the articulated demand is essentially a demand for love.
>
> Desire appears in the rift which separated need and demand; it cannot be reduce to need since, by definition, it is not a relation to a real object independent of the subject but a relation to phantasy; nor can it be reduced to demand, in that it seeks to impose itself without taking the language or the unconscious of the other into account, and upon absolute recognition from him.
>
> (p. 483)

DOI: 10.4324/9781003325314-5

For Lacan, human desire finds its meaning in the desire of the Other, not so much because the Other holds the key to the desired object, but because the first object of human desire is to be recognized by the Other (Lacan, 2020, p. 261). Reworking Hegel's intersubjective formulation of desire within a psychoanalytic framework, the French psychoanalyst argues that the child desires to be desired by the desire of the Other.

As Di Ciaccia and Recalcati (2000) observe,

> To desire the desire of another is, ultimately, to desire that the value that I am, or that I represent, should be the value desired by this other: I want them to recognize my value as their value; I want them to recognize me as an autonomous value. In other words, every human, anthropogenic desire is ultimately a function of the desire for recognition
>
> (p. 169, my translation).

I am aware that the Lacanian theorization of desire may initially appear, on a first reading, as a play on words that is not immediately accessible; nevertheless, in my view it retains considerable clinical and theoretical usefulness. In particular, this perspective allows for a more precise clarification of the distinction between desire and need – a distinction that proves crucial for understanding psychopathological functioning, and especially the dynamics specific to addiction.

If desire is related to the 'lack-of-being'[1] (*manque-à-être*), that is, to a constitutive and structural lack which sets the subject in motion and through which singularity, uniqueness, and individuality are expressed (in the sense that what I desire does not necessarily coincide with what another desires), need (such as hunger or thirst), by contrast, belongs to an eminently bodily register. It manifests as an immediate urgency, as a demand that does not tolerate delay. It does not open a psychic or symbolic space but instead calls for an object capable of eliminating a physiological tension.

The addictive-object is situated precisely within this latter domain. It is not sought because it is desired, but because it is necessary to restore regulation to a disorganized autonomic state. It does not represent what is lacking, but rather what must intervene immediately in order to soothe an unmentalized anxiety, a "nameless dread"[2] (Bion, 1962). The use of the addictive-object therefore does not belong to the economy of desire and does not constitute a creative movement, but rather a compulsive response to a need for safety that does not allow for waiting.

As Jan Winhall (2021) states, addicted patients use

> *addictive behaviours to propel themselves from a state of sympathetic arousal to a dorsal vagal response of numbing, and vice versa. Through understanding how the ANS operates, we see these behaviours as adaptive. They have developed over time to help the addicted person survive when enough safety isn't available*
>
> (p. 4, italics in the original).

From Safety to Desire

In a volume I edited with Clara Mucci, entitled *Embodied Psychoanalysis: Body, Mind and Relationship*, I propose that the drive towards the pursuit of safety is regulated by what I have defined the "principle of safety": a primary bodily necessity which, from a psychodynamic perspective, also involves the psychic domain of the non-repressed unconscious.

What I mean is that, in order for desire to emerge, the primary biological need of the body to register an environment as sufficiently safe must first have been met at an evolutionary level. Once stabilized, this implicit memory translates into a basic sense of safety, both biological and psychological. From this standpoint, the principle of safety represents the precondition for a mode of mental functioning that can be governed by the pleasure principle.

Clinical observation clearly shows how the life of the addicted subject is organized around an incessant attempt to satisfy the need for safety, which comes to override the pleasure principle. For this reason, the first therapeutic task is to help the patient construct, within the therapeutic relationship, a sufficiently stable experience of safety – that is, to allow the patient to feel that, within that space, they can lower their defences without fear of being judged, rejected, or abandoned.

Only from this intersubjective experience does it become possible to orient the therapeutic process towards affect regulation and the development of fragile or underdeveloped mentalizing capacities. This involves supporting the patient in recognizing what is happening within themselves, attributing meaning to it, and finding words to name intense and sometimes violent emotional states that automatically and compulsively drive the dysregulated use of the addictive-object.

These are capacities that, in the histories of such patients, have struggled to be consolidated. When basic safety is lacking, the possibility of experiencing the relationship with oneself and with others in a creative and desirous way is also compromised: the relationship ceases to be a space for exploration and becomes a field of threat – no longer a place where desire can emerge, but an anguishing and painful scenario in which survival becomes the primary concern.

Bodies

Whether one is dealing with desire or with the satisfaction of an urgent need, there is no doubt that the body plays a central role in the development of addictions – not merely as a container of distress. The body enters the consulting room before words, before awareness. It is the body that speaks when the mind falls silent; it is the body that asks for help when affect is too intense to be thought.

In addiction, the substance acts first and foremost on the body, anaesthetizing painful affects and silencing emotions that might otherwise overwhelm the subject. As van der Kolk has taught us, it is always the body that 'keeps the score' of traumatic experiences, preserving their traces even when narrative memory fails. And it is again from the body that every authentic process of healing must inevitably begin.

Yet speaking of *the* body in the singular risks being misleading. Clinical experience clearly shows that what we observe, listen to, and engage with in therapeutic work is never a single, homogeneous body. Rather, the body presents itself through different registers, which intertwine, overlap, or at times come into conflict with one another.

For this reason, it is more appropriate to speak of bodies, distinguishing between the *biological body*, the *affective body*, and the *symbolic body* (Craparo, 2018). These are not abstract categories, but different ways in which the subject inhabits and lives their body. I shall discuss them here in relation to addiction.

The Biological Body

This is the body understood as an organism: the body of organs, neurophysiological systems, genetic vulnerabilities, intoxications, and withdrawals. It is the body that becomes ill, that shows signs of wear, that changes over time, that grows, ages, and declines – a body embedded in an evolutionary history and an environment, bearing features that speak of biological and cultural belonging. In traumatized subjects, it is also the body that carries the scars of years of abuse or neglect, from which it protects itself in order to ensure survival.

It is at this level that instincts operate, understood as relatively specific modes of response to particular environmental stimuli. It is also here that attachment behaviour can be located, understood as an innate disposition towards the search for care. This behaviour is deeply linked to a central characteristic of the human species: *neoteny*. Human beings are born biologically incomplete, fragile, lacking those 'highly specialized organs' that would allow for autonomous survival. This structural fragility renders the presence of the other indispensable and grounds, from the outset, a primary dependency that is not pathological but constitutive.

Neoteny does not concern infancy alone, but extends across the entire lifespan, preserving into adulthood features of plasticity, receptivity, and the need for protective contexts. In this sense, the biological body is never merely nature: it is already profoundly intertwined with culture, family, and the subject's relational history. In many addicted patients, what we observe is precisely a form of suffering that inscribes itself within this original fragility, reactivated and chronically maintained.

The Affective Body

The affective body, or soma, is the felt and lived body, emotionally invested. As Schore (2026) emphasizes, intersubjective relationships are first and foremost relationships between bodies that communicate affects. In the early years of life, the caregiver's body is called upon to attune to the child's body, to contain and modulate states of arousal so that they can gradually be internalized.

When this affective synchronization fails chronically, the body becomes the privileged site of dysregulation: affect – understood as somatic information signalling the level of activation of vital organs – fails to transform into thinkable emotion and subsequently into nameable feeling. In addicted patients, this often manifests as a profound difficulty in recognizing what is happening within themselves, the condition known as alexithymia: "I only feel tension", "I feel bad in my body", "I have to drink to calm down". In such expressions, it is the affective body that speaks, where the mind appears not to have developed reflective capacities sufficient to listen, understand, and consciously name experience.

In the clinical setting, asking the patient what emotion they are feeling invites them to undertake a complex operation: starting from bodily sensations and managing to associate them with an emotion – that is, attributing emotional meaning to bodily experience by linking it to a conscious sensory image, what Edelman (1989) defined as primary or emotional consciousness. Bucci refers to this operation – often compromised in addicted individuals – as *non-verbal symbolic processing*.

The substance thus comes to function as an external regulator of affect, a means by which the subject attempts to silence the body when arousal becomes unbearable, whether excessively high (sympathetic hyperactivation) or drastically reduced (dorsal vagal hypoactivation). From the perspective of relational neurobiology, recourse to the addictive-object can be understood in relation to a structural alteration of the 'window of tolerance', a concept introduced by Daniel J. Siegel (2010) to describe the "band of arousal (of any kind) within an individual can function well" (p. 137).

When the individual remains within this window, the nervous system functions with sufficient regulation to allow simultaneous access to emotions, higher cognitive functions, and relational capacities. In this state, experience can be mentalized, symbolized, and shared without becoming either overwhelming or anaesthetized.

The window of tolerance, however, is not an innate and fixed endowment, but the product of an evolutionary and relational process. It is constructed through early attachment interactions via repeated experiences of affective co-regulation with caregivers. When the caregiver is able to modulate the intensity of the child's emotional states and to accompany them back to equilibrium following moments of activation, the child gradually internalizes this regulatory function, expanding their window of tolerance. The relational environment is then experienced by the autonomic nervous system as sufficiently safe.

By contrast, when activation exceeds the upper limit of the window, the individual enters a state of hyperarousal, characterized by intense anxiety, rage, panic, motor agitation, and loss of control. When activation falls below the lower limit, a state of hypoarousal emerges, marked by withdrawal, numbness, emotional anaesthesia, dissociation, and a sense of emptiness. In both conditions, integration between body, emotion, and thought is compromised.

Siegel emphasizes that trauma – particularly when early and relational in nature – tends to narrow the window of tolerance, rendering the individual vulnerable to rapid and repeated shifts between hyper- and hypoactivation. Addictive behaviour can be understood as an extreme and substitute attempt at self-regulation, aimed at bringing the organism back within a tolerable zone of activation. This form of regulation is rigid, temporary, and dysfunctional: it does not promote the integration of experience, but maintains fragmentation and a dependence on the addictive-object.

For this reason, psychotherapy in such cases cannot be limited to a *talking cure*: it must also – and first and foremost – be a *communicative cure* (Schore, 2015), mediated through embodied affect regulation.

The Symbolic Body

The symbolic body is the body that speaks through language and, in speaking, narrates the subject and their history. It is the thought body, the subjectivized body, capable of transforming experience into representation and metaphor. It is the body that can experience shame and guilt, that can inhabit desire and confront loss.

In clinical practice, when the symptom relates to the symbolic body, it can be translated into a message, a question addressed to the other. In such cases, the body does not merely express distress, but signifies it, inscribing it within a meaningful narrative. When the symbolic body is compromised or fragile, by contrast, the symptom tends to remain a pure signal or discharge, devoid of representational value and therefore unthinkable.

This is precisely what is observed in addiction. Unlike neurotic symptoms, which are structured as symbolic formations or as a language, addictive symptoms are linked to mental disintegration and a failure of symbolization. In other words, in the addicted subject the body often 'communicates' something that lies outside language and meaning: the subject acts, consumes, repeats, where words struggle to emerge and experience remains "unthought known"[3] (Bollas, 1987, p. 213–14).

The Three Bodies in Addiction

In clinical work with addiction, these three bodies are not always simultaneously involved, nor are they necessarily integrated. The patient enters the session bearing a biological body marked by repeated substance use, an affective body often exposed to extreme levels of arousal, and a symbolic body that is fragile, intermittent, or at times almost entirely absent. Affects may impose themselves with an intensity that finds no words; sensation may remain in a raw state, unable to be transformed into emotion or feeling; pain may remain excluded from representation.

When symbolic capacity is sufficiently preserved, the body can become narrative, holding together emotion and the conflict that traverses it, and the symptom may then take the form of a message, a question addressed to the other. When, by contrast, a disintegrated organization prevails – as in addiction – the symptom tends to manifest as discharge, as action that interrupts thought. Therapeutic work is then first and foremost called upon to contain, regulate, and offer an initial possibility of affective holding.

In this sense, treating addiction means working with and through bodies – especially the biological and affective bodies – within a bottom-up therapeutic process, in which the patient becomes familiar with their autonomic nervous system, their sensations and emotions, and their bodily signals. Gradually, sensations can be transformed into thoughts, so that what is today expressed as urgency or repetition may, over time, gain access to symbolization, conscious thought, and speech.

Notes

1 For Lacan, desire is a relation of being to lack. The lack is the lack of being, properly speaking. It isn't the lack of this or that, but the lack of being whereby the being exists. Jacques Lacan's notion of 'lack-of-being' (*manque-à-être*) refers to the constitutive division at the heart of the human subject, which emerges with entry into language and the Symbolic Order, and with the consequent loss of an imagined state of primordial wholeness. This lack is not to be understood as a mere deficit, but as the very condition that gives rise to desire. It sets the subject in motion, sustaining an endless search for a lost object that can never be fully recovered.

Subjectivity is thus formed through processes of alienation, notably in the mirror stage and in the subject's relation to the Big Other – language, culture, and the social order – within which identity takes shape. From this perspective, the human subject is structurally incomplete, defined not by what it possesses but by what it lacks, and perpetually divided between self-image and being. This structural division underlies the dynamics of neurotic striving and the persistent tension that characterizes human desire.

2 "Normal development follows if the relationship between infant and breast permits the infant to project a feeling, say, that it is dying, into the mother and to reintroject it after its sojourn in the breast has made it tolerable to the infant psyche. If the projection is not accepted by the mother the infant feels that its feeling that it is dying is stripped of such meaning as it has. It therefore reintrojects, not a fear of dying made tolerable, but a nameless dread" (Bion, 1962, p. 159)

3 "Refers to any form of knowledge that as yet is not thought. Genetically based knowledge – what constitutes instinctive knowledge – has not been thought out. Infants also learn rules for being and relating that are conveyed though the mother's logic of care, much of which has not been mentally processed. Children often live in family moods or practices that are beyond comprehension, even if they are partners in the living of such knowledge" (Bollas, 1987, pp. 213–14).

Chapter 5

Alexithymia and Addiction

In alexithymic patients, emotional experience tends to remain confined to a bodily and sensory level, without being adequately transformed into shareable mental representations (Taylor, Bagby, & Parker, 1997). In such individuals, a wide range of emotions are not recognized as emotions as such, but are instead lived as undifferentiated somatic states, internal tensions, or physical sensations that are difficult to name. Owing to the impairment of a sufficiently structured symbolic function, the body thus becomes the primary theatre of affective experience, while language tends to be impoverished, concrete, or stereotyped.

The literature distinguishes between trait alexithymia and state alexithymia. The former is described as a relatively stable personality characteristic, structured early within a traumatic developmental context, and capable of constituting a vulnerability factor for the onset and maintenance of various psychiatric disorders. State alexithymia, by contrast, is a transient and reversible condition that emerges in response to intense stress or emotional overload.

From the 1990s onwards, alexithymia attracted increasing interest as a potential predictor of dissociative tendencies (Zlotnick et al., 1996). Dissociation can interfere with the integration of affective, cognitive, and voluntary behavioural control processes, facilitating the development of a split between the physiological, cognitive, and affective components of emotional experience. Both dissociation and alexithymia are considered to contribute to deficits in the perception and processing of emotions, enabling survivors of traumatic experiences to manage affective states that are excessively intense or difficult to tolerate.

According to the theoretical model proposed here, addictive behaviour constitutes a compensatory mode of emotional regulation: the addictive-object intervenes where mentalizing processes fail, offering the immediate modulation of internal states via somato-sensory pathways. The addicted person experiences intense, painful, and overwhelming emotional states in the context of an evolutionary compromise in the capacities to recognize, differentiate, and mentalize emotions, as well as to modulate them effectively (Fonagy et al., 2002).

DOI: 10.4324/9781003325314-6

From this perspective, the triad addiction–dissociation–alexithymia (affect dysregulation) can be understood as a psychopathological constellation signalling a structural vulnerability of personality organization, rooted in early traumatic or severely misattuned relational experiences.

Shame and Narcissistic Rage

If alexithymia signals the difficulty of identifying, differentiating, and communicating emotional states, shame often represents the deepest traumatic affective core: a pervasive, global sense of unworthiness that is frequently dissociated and not always immediately accessible in clinical practice. As Bromberg (2001) emphasizes, shame is closely connected to traumatic memories that compromise the sense of the continuity of the self and of personal value, damaging the possibility of experiencing oneself as intact and recognizable across time.

Because it is generated by experiences that injure self-image, shame forces the subject to see themselves through the gaze of the other, producing a painful rupture between how one feels inwardly and how one imagines one is seen. When such experiences can be recognized and integrated, they contribute to the development of emotional intelligence and open possibilities for self-transformation. When, however, they are denied or dissociated, shame tends to organize itself as a chronic affective state, fostering conditions of generalized anxiety, dysphoria, and mood disturbance, and constituting an important vulnerability factor for the development of addiction.

From an evolutionary–relational perspective, the roots of traumatic shame are often located in experiences of emotional neglect and traumatic attachment during childhood and adolescence. At an implicit level, such experiences may result in hypersensitivity and a vulnerability of the self, facilitating the organization of dissociative functioning aimed at compensating for a structural narcissistic fragility. Clinically, this vulnerability manifests through an inadequate sense of self-efficacy, low self-esteem, disturbed body image, and compromised mentalizing capacities, frequently associated with alexithymic traits.

Judith Lightstone (2004), while referring to different clinical pictures, proposes an understanding of shame as a traumatic affect that is useful for conceptualizing addictive dynamics. From this perspective, addictive behaviour functions as self-medication for shame and intrusive traumatic symptoms, redirecting attention towards the body and the act, and facilitating dissociative processes. Early and traumatic experiences of shame are thereby displaced from the relational domain into the bodily–behavioural domain, assuming a form that is more tolerable and, in some respects, more 'acceptable' than their relational origin, which has by then become dissociated.

This reading is fully consistent with Bromberg's (2001) hypotheses, according to which addicted patients appear overwhelmed by physiological and affective states because, throughout development, they have lacked sufficiently reliable interpersonal experience capable of repairing frustrations and supporting the regulation of affects and desires. The traumatic component of primary relational experience is dissociated and re-emerges in the form of a psychopathology in which the relationship with the addictive-object implicitly represents early object relations, characterized by discontinuity, unpredictability, and unreliability.

Developing these hypotheses further, one might argue that the addicted subject remains trapped in impulsive–compulsive behaviour precisely because it allows for the denial of the interpersonal desire for the protection of the self. This dynamic can be described as a form of narcissistic self-sufficiency, through which the individual attempts to heal self-wounds by displaying a renunciation of the other and of their relational needs. This defence, however, inevitably collides with the self's imperfections and with internal objects derived from neglectful childhood relationships, fuelling an increasingly intense spiral of shame and narcissistic rage. Shame and rage are the two emotions with which the clinician most often contends in the treatment of traumatized/addicted patients.

As Kohut (1971) observed, the most intense experiences of shame and narcissistic rage emerge in those individuals for whom the maintenance of self-esteem depends crucially on the unconditional availability of the self-object and on control of the environment.

The shame–narcissistic rage dyad thus reflects a profound difficulty in coming into contact with one's feelings. The dissociative practices implicated in addiction are involved in the attempt to anaesthetize the body and the experience of violent emotions to which the addicted person is continuously exposed.

In therapeutic work, it is essential to support the patient in recovering traumatic emotions so that they can be processed. This presupposes the construction of a strong therapeutic alliance and a setting experienced as a secure base (Bowlby, 1988), within which the patient can gradually gain access to their narcissistic destructiveness, give words to shame, and undertake a process of self-integration, progressively reducing the need for the regulatory function of addiction.

Shame and Rage in the Therapeutic Setting

Shame may manifest itself explicitly, when the patient reports directly feeling ashamed in the presence of others; more often, however, it tends to appear within the therapeutic field through interactive configurations. In the clinical setting, it may emerge in the form of prolonged silences, relational withdrawal, sudden discontinuities in narrative, compulsive behaviour, oscillations between the idealization and devaluation of the therapist, as well as a marked difficulty in tolerating the other's gaze, recognition, and emotional closeness.

The patient does not name shame as such but speaks of profound feelings of unworthiness; they express the conviction that, should someone come too close, that person would be horrified and disgusted, and they fear being seen in their presumed unacceptability. For this reason, for these patients it is difficult to be seen without being humiliated, welcomed without being invaded, or recognized without being exposed.

A clinical example may clarify these dynamics. Michele, a 35-year-old man with a long history of marijuana and alcohol dependence, enters therapy complaining of emptiness, impulsivity, and frequent relapses, yet without being able to recognize or name specific emotional states. During the initial sessions, he tends to provide detailed and concrete accounts of his behaviours, systematically avoiding any reference to the affective dimension. Any attempt by the therapist to approach the underlying emotional experience is met with sudden silences, lowered gaze, or devaluing comments directed at the treatment itself. Only over time does it become clear that these reactions are associated with an intense, unspoken experience of shame, linked to the perception of being seen as weak, dependent, and morally inadequate. In this context, addiction appears to serve an anaesthetizing function and a somatic regulation of a painful affective state, enabling the patient to withdraw from the relational experience of shame through recourse to the addictive-object.

Giovanna is a 49-year-old woman who enters therapy following the end of a romantic relationship. She speaks of her former partner in strongly devaluing terms, describing him as unreliable and dishonest and defining him, in highly aggressive language, as “a piece of shit, the biggest piece of shit in the city”. From the first sessions, an intense affective activation emerges, in which rage occupies a central place and appears to obstruct any reflective processing of experience.

Over the course of treatment, deeper relational experiences gradually surface, marked by an inner tear linked to severely dysfunctional parental figures. Her father, who died around ten years earlier, is described as cold, violent towards her and her mother, and as a serial betrayer. When Giovanna speaks of him, she appears visibly agitated; the narrative is permeated by intense rage, ferociously expressed, which seems to overwhelm thought.

She also reports a persistent difficulty sustaining stable interpersonal relationships, particularly with men. Since adolescence, she has lived with a constant fear of becoming attached to a violent, deceitful, and unfaithful partner (traits of the father), a fear that, in her experience, tends to be repeatedly confirmed. This relational repetition can be understood as a re-enactment of early internal working models characterized by unpredictability, danger, and lack of reliability, which organize her object choices and affective dynamics.

Her relationship with her mother has also always been complex and ambivalent. Towards her, Giovanna feels a mixture of pity and reproach for not leaving her husband and for having allowed both herself and her daughter to endure that man’s violence. In describing her mother’s character traits, a markedly depressive picture emerges, evocative of Green's (1993) “dead mother complex”,[1] in which the maternal presence appears affectively withdrawn, unable to offer adequate support or to perform a function of emotional mirroring.

The patient's family and relational history is accompanied by a deep and pervasive conviction of being unworthy of being desirable in the eyes of the other. This experience also emerges in dream material. In one dream, Giovanna reports having intercourse with her father; as she recounts it, her body becomes rigid and her expression conveys disgust and contempt. More than lending itself to an Oedipal reading, the dream in fact points to a relational modality in which the other's sexual investment is accompanied by immediate withdrawal, driven by fear of intimacy and by the reactivation of traumatic experiences of shame and contamination. This dynamic frequently expresses itself through fierce devaluation of the self or the other. Particularly significant is Giovanna's comment after having had the dream: "I'm rotten inside" – an expression of a profound sense of unworthiness and of a self experienced as intrinsically damaged.

This affective core intertwines with a long history of substance use. Since adolescence, Giovanna has consumed significant amounts of alcohol, with episodes of cocaine use primarily at weekends. Substance use appears closely connected to intense and difficult-to-tolerate emotional states, functioning as a mode of affect regulation and containment of painful internal states, particularly rage and shame.

I have included these two clinical vignettes to highlight the importance of therapeutic work initially focusing on maintaining a stable, predictable, and non-judgemental relational stance, capable of containing oscillations between withdrawal and compulsive behaviour, between devaluation and idealization. Only when the patient begins to experience the setting as sufficiently safe does an initial reflective access to shame and rage become possible – affects that can gradually be named and linked to early relational experiences of humiliation and emotional neglect. In this way, these two affects progressively lose their dissociative and totalizing quality, reducing the need for the regulatory function of an external object and opening the way towards a more stable and articulated process of self-integration.

Note

1 For Arnold H. Modell (1999) it is useful to distinguish the dead mother *complex* from the dead mother *syndrome*: "The term dead mother syndrome can be used to denote the intensely malignant clinical syndrome that Green described when there is a primary identification with the emotionally dead mother whereas the term dead mother complex denotes an entire range of an individual's response to a chronically depressed, emotionally absent mother" (p. 76).

Chapter 6

Trauma, Dissociation, and Addiction

Starting with Pierre Janet, psychopathological and neuroscientific research on trauma has progressively clarified the profound link between trauma and dissociation (Janet, 1889; van der Kolk, 2014; Howell, 2020; van der Hart, 2024; Porges, 2021; Schore, 2015). These contributions converge in affirming that trauma is not simply remembered but remains encapsulated within bodily memory. The traumatized patient is, first and foremost, a body that is sensitive to threat, constantly prepared to respond defensively. The problem is that this state of alert tends never to switch off.

Traumatized individuals thus remain bound to a past of neglect, abuse or maltreatment that continues to be re-enacted, with a marked difficulty in remaining anchored in the present. In Giovanna's case, for example, it was sufficient to observe her body language to grasp the reactivation of trauma. The patient appeared anchored, on a sensory and emotional level – but also at an unconscious level – to a past that profoundly and pervasively shaped her perception of herself and others, her thoughts, her feelings, her fantasies, and her expectations of a future that she imagined as an endless repetition of what had already been lived.

This view of the world, of the self, and of the future is the expression of a traumatic bond: a past that does not pass and that continues to return. A repetition that runs across generations – parents, relatives – and that has ultimately organized Giovanna's personal history as well, keeping her imprisoned within a traumatic continuity that struggles to find a path towards transformation.

But what do we mean by the term trauma? This is not a trivial question, given that the literature does not appear to offer a unanimous definition. In the DSM (2013, 2022), trauma is described in relation to the intrinsic characteristics of the event, largely excluding personal dimensions. Some authors speak of positive trauma, while others distinguish between trauma (with a lowercase t) and Trauma (with an uppercase T).

Beyond the different theoretical positions present in the literature, there seems to be at least one point of agreement: trauma is always something that is harmful to the individual's physical and psychological equilibrium.

DOI: 10.4324/9781003325314-7

Over the years, I have developed the idea – shared by other colleagues – that, rather than being understood primarily in relation to the intrinsic characteristics of the event (which does not mean that these should be disregarded), trauma should be conceptualized starting from subjective experience and from the emotional impact that one or more events exert on the individual's somatopsychic balance.

Before examining the influence of these factors in the process of traumatization, it is, in my view, necessary to clarify the relationship between trauma and stress.

From Stress to Traumatic Stress

The term stress is now widely used in everyday language to describe situations that require significant emotional and cognitive engagement, prompting us to find strategies capable of restoring psychophysical balance.

Etymologically, stress means tension, and it may manifest with varying intensity in response to everyday situations such as preparing for a university examination or a job interview, obtaining a desired position, or waiting for an important meeting, as well as to more emotionally impactful events such as illness, bereavement, a road traffic accident, having witnessed a homicide, or events that profoundly compromise personal dignity and integrity, such as abuse, neglect or maltreatment perpetrated by significant figures or strangers.

It is undeniable that the impact of a stressor – here I will explicitly refer to the pathological manifestations of stress – varies from person to person. A violent experience, for example, may be experienced as extremely overwhelming by one individual, while for another it may have a less intense and more transient resonance. The differing psychophysical effects of stress depend not only on the nature of the event that elicited it, its duration, and whether it is an isolated episode or repeated over time, but also – and above all – on variables related to the person, such as age, personal history, physical health status, cognitive and emotional resources, coping strategies, internalized attachment style, the presence or absence of social support, as well as genetic factors.

When we consider trauma from the perspective of the individual, we tend to distinguish *non-traumatic stress* from *traumatic stress* (or trauma). The former is generally classified into two main forms: acute and chronic. Acute stress manifests immediately during or shortly after a stressful event. It is characterized by transience and a lack of pervasiveness, although in some cases it may have a significant psychophysical impact, to the point of evolving into a clinical condition such as acute stress disorder. Chronic stress, by contrast, persists over time and manifests across different areas of the person's life, compromising their choices and psychophysical wellbeing, at least until it is adequately addressed. An example of the psychopathological development of chronic stress is post-traumatic stress disorder.

Resilience to stress – that is, the capacity to manage adequately the effects of emotionally stressful events – depends on a range of constitutional, psychological, medical, and social factors specific to the individual. This means that resilience is not the same for everyone. Some people are able to process a stressful event, while others remain caught up in it, unable to find a way out or an effective solution. For all of us, the first step of resilience consists in survival. Traumatized patients, as noted, develop survival strategies that are so refined that they become bound by them, to the point of being unable to make space for a fully lived life, animated by interaction and secure connection with the environment. Rather than living, they are constantly engaged in attempting to protect themselves from an environment perceived – and neuroceived (Porges, 2011) – as threatening, even in the absence of any real danger.

With regard to the incidence of personal variables in stress management, it is useful to revisit the rope metaphor proposed by Tracey Shors (2021):

> It helps to think of each person as a rope. One person might be born with a strong, thick rope, while another is born with a thin, more fragile one. Someone who ended up with PTSD after 9/11 might have been born with a more fragile rope or lived through circumstances that frayed the rope, making it more vulnerable even before that day. If you have a stronger rope or can cultivate one, it will take more stress to break it. But if you have a fragile one or if life has weakened your rope along the way, a smaller amount of stress can cause it to fray and maybe even break. We can make our ropes stronger with healthy behaviours, such as physical exercise, eating well, and sleeping well. But we should also go beyond the obvious. We can train our brains to learn new skills that will help us accept and live with our own thoughts and memories – more on how to do this later. Then, when stress and trauma arise, our ropes will be less likely to break
>
> (p. 3).

In traumatized patients, the rope has not merely frayed; it has snapped. This metaphor highlights the fundamental difference between non-traumatic stress and traumatic stress. In the former case, the individual experiences a condition of persistent tension that generates psychological and somatic suffering and may evolve into a psychopathological picture. However, the ventral-vagal social engagement system is not completely deactivated, meaning that the sense of safety, although compromised, is not entirely absent.

By contrast, traumatic stress – or trauma – is characterized by a profound internal rupture, namely a structural dissociation that keeps the individual in a constant state of insecurity and a pervasive need for protection. In this condition, the social engagement system is deactivated, and the person lives in a persistent psychophysical state of alert, accompanied by dissociative symptoms.

Trauma may therefore be understood as the result of a deep wound, associated with one or more 'breaking points' (Ross, 1941) involving both body and mind.

From this perspective, trauma is indissolubly linked to dissociation: not only does a relationship exist between trauma and dissociation, but trauma is itself dissociative. In my view, without this internal fracture, we could not identify a patient as traumatized.

Dissociative Trauma

The close relationship between trauma and dissociation outlined in the previous section has led me to formulate the construct of dissociative trauma (Craparo, 2026). The term dissociative refers both to structural dissociation, associated with the internal wound/fracture generated by one or more emotionally overwhelming events, and to dissociation as a defensive mechanism, as well as to the associated psychopathological outcomes.

Speaking of dissociative trauma reinforces the idea that it is not solely events in themselves that are traumatic, but rather the subjective experience that determines their impact. This means that an event such as abuse may become a traumatic experience in relation, as noted above, to a compromise in the victim's capacities for processing and mentalization.

As Chefetz (2015) argues:

> Traumatic experience has occurred when there has been a sudden or cumulative experience that alters the developmental trajectory of an individual through changes in the organization or constitution of their self-states, the ability to have emotional experience, the capacity to think and balance associative and dissociative processes, the capacity to live in relationship with self and others, and the maintenance of an enduring sense of self, all of which is reflected in alterated neurobiological function
>
> (p. 191).

In this passage, Chefetz highlights how the impact of a stressful event on psychological and physical health cannot be understood independently of the individual's developmental and relational history. From this perspective, dissociative trauma represents a distinctive element that emerges in response to emotionally overwhelming experiences, perceived as threatening or dangerous to the person's somatopsychic survival, and that may lead to a disaggregation of subjective experience and of personality organization.

The degree and intensity of such traumatic experiences do not depend exclusively on the intrinsic characteristics of the event or on its frequency, but are strongly modulated by biological, psychological and relational factors.

Biological Factors

With regard to biological factors, clinical and neuroscientific research has progressively highlighted how vulnerability to dissociative trauma cannot be attributed solely to the nature of the traumatic event, but rather emerges from the complex interaction between individual predispositions and the environmental context. Several studies have identified a hereditary component in the development of trauma-related disorders, such as post-traumatic stress disorder (Duncan, Cooper & Shen, 2018), suggesting that some individuals may exhibit greater biological sensitivity to stressful events.

In parallel, growing interest has focused on the processes through which the relational environment and early traumatic experiences may modulate gene expression via epigenetic mechanisms. This line of research has shown that stressful events – particularly when chronic and relational in nature – can produce stable biological modifications, influencing stress-response systems and, in some cases, becoming transmissible across generations. From this perspective, trauma is no longer conceived as a time-limited event, but as an experience capable of leaving enduring traces in the body, thereby contributing to an understanding of the long-term and transgenerational effects of traumatic suffering.

From a neurophysiological standpoint, it is now well established that traumatic stress and dissociative trauma are associated with profound alterations in the systems responsible for the protection and regulation of the organism. These alterations may manifest as changes in neuroendocrine and immune functioning. Clinical studies have shown, for example, dysregulation of the hypothalamic–pituitary–adrenal (HPA) axis and alterations in immune system functioning in individuals exposed to childhood and/or adult trauma (Ramo-Fernández et al., 2015), suggesting that such changes may exert long-lasting effects on stress responsiveness and increase vulnerability to physical illness.

Within this framework, Stephen Porges' Polyvagal Theory (2011) offers a particularly useful lens through which to understand the neurobiological processes underlying trauma. According to this model, the autonomic nervous system is not organized merely along a dichotomous axis of activation and relaxation, but rather according to a hierarchy of neurophysiological states that are activated as a function of the perception – often unconscious – of safety or danger in the environment. This process automatically shapes the individual's emotional, behavioural, and relational responses, outside reflective awareness.

Under conditions of perceived safety, activation of the ventral vagal system supports states of calm, relational openness, and affective co-regulation. By contrast, when the environment is experienced as threatening or unpredictable, the organism may resort to more primitive defensive modes: sympathetic–adrenal mobilization, associated with fight-or-flight responses, or dorsal vagal immobilization, which manifests clinically as freezing or collapse. These responses do not represent mere bodily reactions, but rather constitute genuine states of being, profoundly influencing emotional experience, behaviour, and the capacity to remain in relationship with others.

According to polyvagal theory, trauma is fundamentally linked to a chronic dysfunction of autonomic circuits that keeps the individual in a persistent state of hyperarousal or defensive shutdown, thereby hindering affect regulation, mentalization and attachment processes. In this sense, traumatic experience quite literally 'remains in the body', organizing automatic response patterns that dysfunctionally shape how the person perceives themselves, others, and the world.

Psychological Factors

With regard to psychological factors, an area of particular interest is represented by research on personality traits. In particular, the trait of neuroticism has been found to be associated with greater vulnerability to the development of post-traumatic symptoms (Breslau & Schultz, 2013; Ogle et al., 2013), as well as with an increased risk of exposure to overwhelming stressors over the course of the lifespan (Schemitsch & Nauth, 2019).

Other relevant psychological factors concern the use of dysfunctional coping strategies, which may compromise resilience and facilitate the onset of post-traumatic symptoms. In this respect, Pineles et al. (2011) identified a significant association between avoidant coping strategies and the severity of PTSD symptomatology. Morrison and Benight (2022), by contrast, explored the role of self-efficacy in trauma management (Trauma Coping Self-Efficacy), identifying it as a crucial mediator in the relationship between insecure adult attachment and post-traumatic symptoms.

A further psychological factor is mentalization. Several studies confirm that trauma is significantly and negatively correlated with the level of mentalization maturity, in the sense that the more intense the trauma, the less mature the capacity for mentalization, and vice versa. This construct may be understood as a bridging concept between attachment theory, the psychoanalytic tradition and affective neuroscience. It offers an integrated perspective on how cognition and emotion are articulated in the development of the self, and on how adequate social and emotional development protects the individual, whereas trauma compromises the capacity to face pain and suffering in an adaptive manner.

Mentalization does not concern merely the awareness of thoughts and beliefs, but rather the process through which the brain becomes mind, that is, the capacity to represent one's own and others' mental states. From this perspective, mentalization is intrinsically relational: being mentalized by a significant other – first and foremost the caregiver – stimulates the development of the capacity to mentalize the self.

Two elements characterize mentalization: on the one hand, its roots in emotional experience and within the attachment context; on the other, the fact that it concerns both understanding others and the relationship with oneself. The development of mentalization is in fact closely linked to the quality of early attachment relationships, which offer the child not only security, but also the opportunity to recognize mental states as distinct from external reality.

According to Fonagy and Target (1997), affect regulation constitutes the foundation of mentalization; at the same time, mentalization enables more evolved and differentiated forms of emotional regulation, defined as mentalized affectivity. This form of regulation is not limited to the modulation of affects, but entails the capacity to attribute meaning to emotional experience, integrating it into autobiographical memory and personal history. For Jurist (2005), the term mentalized affectivity describes a process that includes the identification, processing and expression of affects, allowing the individual to tolerate and think about emotions rather than acting impulsively upon them. Mentalization and mentalized affectivity represent not only a developmental goal, but also a central therapeutic factor, particularly in the treatment of trauma, where the capacity to think about emotions becomes an essential condition for interrupting repetition and promoting integration of the self.

Social Factors

It is widely documented that the absence of a supportive social network constitutes an additional risk factor, negatively affecting the capacity to process emotionally the impact of stressful and potentially traumatic events, as well as contributing to the development of post-traumatic symptomatology.

In the case of neglectful primary relationships, the perception that seeking help may entail shame or lead to an irreparable rupture in family bonds can become unbearable. In such circumstances, beyond the nature of the event itself, what proves devastating is the response – often inadequate, ambiguous, or hostile – of the attachment environment, which ideally should offer protection, validation, and containment.

One of my patients, who was sexually abused by her maternal grandfather at the age of 15, found the courage to confide in her mother. Instead of receiving understanding and support, however, her mother accused her of lying, reproached her by saying that such 'fantasies' risked ruining both herself and the entire family, and ordered her not to tell her father for fear that he might 'lose his head' and attack the grandfather. This response constituted a double shock: to the abuse suffered was added denial and betrayal by the primary attachment figure.

Not being believed and being unable to rely on family support – on which the patient depended, but which was simultaneously a source of threat – triggered a profound malaise that evolved into a severe depressive state and self-harming behaviours.

How many cases of violence and abuse have remained hidden, leaving victims (often women) alone to bear a burden that exceeded their capacities, draining them of vitality and, in some cases, driving them to suicide as a final solution to a harm experienced as profoundly unjust and oppressive?

Discrimination, poverty, war, and social isolation can be experiences so intensely stressful as to provoke, in some cases, the emergence of psychopathological conditions linked to traumatic stress (dissociative trauma).

If the absence of social support can allow trauma to sediment, experiences of solidarity and a willingness to receive and hold the pain of a suffering or traumatized person constitute the very foundations of a civil society, in which being human means not abandoning those who cry out in their loneliness and pain.

Developmental–Relational Factors

It should now be clear that when I speak of trauma, I do not distinguish it from what is non-traumatic on the basis of the objective nature of the event – as occurs in the DSM-5 (2013) – but rather by considering the processes and structures that, from the earliest years of life, influence the individual's psychic and somatic functioning (Schore, 2012; Craparo, 2013; Mucci, 2018).

By integrating attachment studies, affective neuroscience research, and investigations into developmental stress, Allan Schore (2001, 2013) found that children who experienced abuse in the first two years of life and traumatic attachment relationships with caregivers are frequently unable to develop functional and adaptive strategies for coping with relational stress. According to Schore, traumatic attachments experienced from the earliest years of life and throughout development negatively affect right-brain development and, consequently, emotional regulation and coping mechanisms, both mental and physical, rendering the individual more vulnerable to the development of symptoms associated with dissociative trauma.

Within this framework, the crucial role of failures in emotional attunement between parent and child comes into focus. Attunement refers to the sensitive capacity to grasp and recognize another person's emotional world. It does not simply coincide with parental love. A parent may deeply love their child and be highly protective, yet still fail to attune to the child's emotional needs (as in cases of parental overprotection), just as occurs in situations of emotional neglect.

A lack of attunement on the part of the caregiver may foster in the child a sense of not being truly seen, of not being recognized in their subjectivity: the implicit message the child may internalize is that of a presence unable to come into contact with their inner world.

This is an extremely delicate process. A frightened or frightening parent, overwhelmed by stress, depressed or affected by a personality disorder may, often unconsciously, absorb and colonize the child's emotional world, depriving them of the opportunity to develop a private inner space and a sense of personal subjectivity. It is in such contexts that the child may come to identify with the emotionally non-attuned parent, developing what has been conceptualized as an internal saboteur.

As Lingiardi (2025) observes,

> Instead of having his or her mental state adequately mirrored, [the child] is forced to internalize the mental state of the abusive parent, which becomes a non-integrated and alien part of the self, the repository of the aggressor's cruelty and of the attempt to manage it through identification (p. 112, my translation).

Over time, this lack of attunement may translate into a profound sense of loneliness or emptiness, or into states of boredom, anger, shame, or depression that are difficult to regulate. Relationships characterized by poor attunement do not provide a sufficiently solid ground for the development of neurological and psychological self-regulation systems. The child is thus forced to find, alone and prematurely, strategies to cope with intense emotional states, laying the foundations for adaptive patterns that may later crystallize into dysfunctional forms.

Within this framework, the process of affective attunement (Stern, 1985) represents a pivotal point in the development of attachment. It is through attunement that the child can communicate needs, begin to distinguish the inner world from external reality, and experience an empathic response from the caregiver. When this regulatory exchange is sufficiently stable, the sense of safety is strengthened: positive emotional states are amplified, while negative ones are modulated and contained. Over time, this regulated alternation allows for the construction of a sense of continuity of the self, enabling the child to move through different emotional experiences without fragmentation.

From this perspective, traumatic attachment may be understood as the internalized product of repeated childhood experiences in which the child felt rejected, neglected or frightened by those who should have guaranteed closeness, protection and emotional regulation. I consider this form of attachment to be closely linked to dissociative trauma. As Felicity de Zulueta et al. (2025) emphasize, traumatic attachment entails an intrinsic dissociative condition (Bowlby, 1980), characterized by the coexistence of separate mental states: at a conscious level, the child maintains an idealized image of the parent, while at a less conscious level there persists a conflicting representation in which the caregiver is experienced as rejecting, neglectful, or abusive.

For Bowlby, the dissociation between these representations serves a fundamental survival need: the protection of the attachment bond. While this solution allows the child to cope with an emotionally frightening condition, it comes at a high cost. The dissociative exclusion of the frightening caregiver from conscious awareness leaves a lasting imprint on relational functioning, exposing the individual in adulthood to a disadvantage in interpersonal relationships compared to those in whom such exclusion is less pronounced.

From a clinical perspective, we know how crucial the capacity to attune to the other's mind is for the maturation of brain systems responsible for affect regulation (Beebe & Lachmann, 2002; Schore, 1994), as well as for the development of social competencies, autobiographical memory, reflective function and narrative processes (Fonagy & Target, 1997; Main, 1995). It is within attuned relationships that the child learns not only to feel, but to make sense of what is felt.

Early experiences of reciprocity foster the integration of different emotional response systems – neurophysiological, behavioural–expressive and cognitive–experiential. When such integration is possible, emotions can be transformed into feelings, that is, into meaningful, modulable and communicable experiences. When attunement fails, as occurs in insecure and traumatic attachment relationships, the child experiences a fracture between the different levels of emotional experience (de Zulueta et al., 2025). This fracture manifests as a deficit in cognitive and metacognitive functions involved in affect processing, accompanied by a disconnection between physiological, behavioural, and experiential levels. Emotions thus cease to function as motivational signals and guides for action, becoming instead sources of confusion or overload.

Concluding Considerations

As stated, the traumatized patient bears the marks of trauma not only in the psyche but also in the body, where traumatic memories become sedimented. This is a traumatized body: a body that retains the memory of somatic responses elicited by adverse events experienced as overwhelming relative to the capacities for processing and integrating the self.

In the previous chapter, I proposed three dimensions of the body (biological, affective, and symbolic): the biological body oriented towards survival; the affective body oriented towards emotional and relational communication; and the symbolic body, understood as the body that expresses itself through language, the body capable of speaking (consciously and unconsciously) to the Other. These three bodies are dynamically intertwined and inseparable from their reciprocal relationship with the psychic sphere, to the extent that one may speak of an embodied psyche.

I believe that these three bodily registers can be related to Wilma Bucci's (1997) multiple code model, according to which affective experience can proceed through two information-processing systems: verbal and non-verbal. The former concerns symbolic processing that can be communicated and shared through language. In Bucci's theorization, language constitutes the code of communication and reflection through which private and subjective experience – including emotional experience – can be shared with others; at the same time, it is the means through which cultural knowledge and logical rules contribute to the construction of individual thought content.

Language is also the code we rely on to orient and self-regulate, to activate imagination and emotions, to stimulate action and to exercise control over it. The verbal code functions predominantly as a single-channel, sequential processor: generally, we are able to produce or comprehend only one verbal message at a time. Finally, language is primarily – though not exclusively – dominant in the state of consciousness.

With regard to the non-verbal system, it includes both sensory–motor forms (non-verbal sub-symbolic) and the processing of information in sensory images (non-verbal symbolic). Within the framework of multiple code theory, emotions are conceived as image–action schemas that may operate both within and outside consciousness.

In general terms, emotional schemas consist of desires, expectations, and beliefs about the self and others, which develop through interpersonal interactions from the very earliest phases of life. These schemas include representations of objects, parts of objects, and the relationships between them across all sensory modalities, together with patterns of activation associated with motor actions and visceral and somatic states.

They therefore encompass images of the object and of emotion – for example, the person we desire, love, or fear – as well as representations, at the level of the central nervous system, of the specific actions linked to emotional activation (such as approach, attack, or flight). Added to this are the patterns of visceral and somatic experiences connected to such activation, that is, what we feel – or expect to feel – in the body, for instance when we are angry, frightened, or in love.

Emotional schemas begin to form within the non-verbal system prior to language acquisition; only at a later stage of development, Bucci argues, can their content be progressively linked to language and symbolic representations.

Within this interpretative model, we can observe that not all patients are able to access a symbolic register of bodily representations (the symbolic body). In the case of addicted patients, this represents a structural impossibility linked to a disaggregation of the self and a consequent impairment of mentalization capacities. In these patients, the traumatic emotions involved in the addictive process remain at a non-verbal sub-symbolic or non-verbal symbolic level, failing to gain access to the symbolic–verbal level.

How can all this be integrated with what I have written about dissociative trauma? First and foremost, by not separating trauma from traumatized patients, who have been exposed to stimuli neuroceived by the biological body as threatening or extremely threatening to survival and physical integrity, eliciting particularly intense emotional reactions (involving the affective body in addition to the biological one). In such individuals, sensorimotor and emotional states have not been processed at a symbolic–verbal level and therefore remain dissociated as unformulated experiences within the unrepressed unconscious (Craparo, 2017; 2018; 2026), *enacted* automatically and repetitively. These enactments are reactivations (*re-enactments*) of dissociated traumatic memories, in which both the disorganizing effects of traumatic emotions and associated sensations, and the survival responses adopted by the biological body, emerge.

The central problem is that these patients remain biologically, emotionally, and psychically trapped in a frightening past from which they are unable to free themselves. They are thus compelled to live in a perpetual state of alert, perceiving reality as threatening, unjust, and dangerous, and feeling the need to defend themselves constantly.

Clinically, this condition manifests in various forms: behavioural hypervigilance, muscular rigidity, bodily tension, exaggerated controlling attitudes, or, conversely, experiences of bodily disconnection, asthenia, and marked disorganization of thought and language, often oriented in a defensive and self-protective manner. Recurrent verbal expressions such as "The world is dangerous", "I can't trust anyone", "I have to protect myself", and "If I let my guard down, anxiety will overwhelm me" reflect the traumatized individual's internal configuration, centred on a bodily and mental state of constant alarm and relational mistrust.

The predominant emotional states in these patients – such as anger, anxiety, anguish, depression, helplessness, loneliness, emptiness, shame, guilt, fear, and boredom – express a psychic functioning that struggles to distinguish between past and present, between safety and real danger.

Chapter 7

Traumatic Attachment Identification

As a psychoanalyst, I cannot avoid considering the role of traumatic identification. By this expression I refer to a process through which traumatic experience – especially when it occurs within significant relationships – is internalized and becomes a constitutive part of the organization of the self. It is not simply a matter of remembering a painful event, but of incorporating its affective, relational and defensive dynamics, to the point that they begin to function as implicit models of perception and of relating to oneself and to others.

In early and chronic interpersonal traumas – particularly in traumatic attachments – the child is exposed to an unbearable contradiction: the caregiver is both a source of protection and a source of threat. In order to survive this contradiction, the child's mind resorts to dissociative solutions that allow the bond to be preserved, even at the cost of sacrificing the integration of self-experience. Traumatic identification consists precisely in the internalization and identification of the traumatic states (internal objects) – relational modes, gaze, violence, emotional withdrawal – of the parent, which coincide with dissociated parts of the self. Given the centrality of traumatic attachment, I propose using the expression *Traumatic Attachment Identification* as a specific articulation of traumatic identification. TAI designates an unconscious (unrepressed) identificatory process that emerges in the context of early relational trauma, when the attachment relationship with the primary figure is simultaneously necessary and threatening. Under such circumstances, the traumatic bond is internalized as an organizing principle of self-experience.

This is a form of identification that guarantees the continuity of attachment at the expense of self-integration, configuring a dissociative organization that, over time, is associated with difficulties in affect regulation, identity coherence and relational functioning.

This identification does not serve a symbolic or representational function, but is predominantly implicit and embodied. It manifests through dissociated self-states, bodily postures, modes of affective activation and deep convictions – often not verbalized – that organize subjective experience.

DOI: 10.4324/9781003325314-8

Thus, a child who has been abused or rejected may, in adulthood, find themselves treating their partner in the same way they were treated by the caregiver, perceiving the other as inevitably threatening or untrustworthy, or reproducing the interpersonal dynamics of submission, control or withdrawal. I am reminded of Janny, a forty-three-year-old patient who, after growing up with a cynical and violent father, found herself as an adult choosing – without being able to understand why – partners who were similarly violent and narcissistic. In her intimate relationships, the same script seemed always to repeat itself: men who were initially seductive, then progressively devaluing, aggressive and intrusive. It was as though Janny were unconsciously driven to re-enact, in the present, the traumatic dynamics she had lived within her original family context – dynamics that did not merely inhabit conscious memory, but had remained imprinted in bodily memory, in her ways of reacting, of attaching, of tolerating abuse, and even of confusing violence with intimacy.

Some authors, such as Correale (2010), define this tendency to re-actualize overwhelming past experiences unconsciously with the term *traumatophilia*: traumatic parts of the self, charged with unmentalized affects and dissociated emotional states, are unconsciously placed in the other (for instance, from parent to child), who comes to embody, within the current relationship, the same figures and persecutory functions of the past. In this way, what has not been symbolized does not remain confined to the past, but returns as lived, enacted and repeated experience.

Traumatophilia, however, is not manifested solely in partner choice. We also find it in self-harming behaviours, addictions, and in all those forms of conduct that appear oriented towards self-destruction – towards sabotaging any possibility of change and openness to a different existence. It is as though the subject remained bound to an internal script in which suffering represents the only known territory and, paradoxically, the only one in which they feel 'at home'. In these repetitions, it is not pain as such that is sought, but the familiarity of a traumatic experience that continues to organize the relationship with oneself, with others and with one's own life.

In *Confusion of Tongues Between Adults and the Child*, Ferenczi (1949) offers an opportunity to better understand these dynamics. Describing the tendency of the maltreated child to regulate fear through identification with the aggressor, Ferenczi argues that:

> *The same anxiety, however, if it reaches a certain maximum, compels them to subordinate themselves like automata to the will of the aggressor, to divine each one of his desires and to gratify these; completely oblivious of themselves they identify themselves with the aggressor.* Through the identification, or let us say, introjection of the aggressor, he disappears as part of the external reality, and becomes intra- instead of extra-psychic; the intra-psychic is then subjected, in a dream-like state as is the traumatic trance, to the primary process, i.e. according to the pleasure principle it

> can be modified or changed by the use of positive or negative hallucinations. In any case the attack as a rigid external reality ceases to exist and in the traumatic trance the child succeeds in maintaining the previous situation of tenderness
>
> (p. 228).

As Cesare Albasi (2006) underlines, the precondition for identification with the aggressor is the dissociation of one's own feelings and perceptions; this process leaves an internal 'void' that is filled by a form of intelligence that is permanently vigilant and oriented towards constantly anticipating the other's will.

In *Borderline Bodies*, Clara Mucci (2018) further develops the theme of identification with the aggressor in order to understand the aggressive and self-destructive behaviours of victims of abuse. The author writes:

> These negative parts internalized as parts of the m/other or of the caregiver … might also be 'externalized' onto the body of others, when aggressiveness is egosyntonic, in connection with a very weak capacity for empathy, which in turn means that the regulation-attachment system with the caregiver has not fostered the appropriate level of self-love, self-esteem, empathy, and regulation. As a consequence, the body becomes the hatred target, either one's body (with masochistic mechanisms rooted in guilt and self-hatred or self-loathing) or the body of the others, through violence directed against the others and society, to the point of criminality and antisocial behaviour. Contrary to an innate view of violence, I see the root of that violence as stemming always from an internalized destructiveness that has been intergenerationally received and relationally internalized through a victim-persecutor model […] this is, in my opinion, the major mechanism of destructiveness and symptom formation in personality disorders.
>
> The mechanism of identification of self and body with 'victim' and self and body with 'persecutor' is a consequence of the introjection of negative affects that result from relational traumatization and abuse
>
> (pp. 20–21).

I agree with this reading, and I would add a further element to understand the paradoxical search for suffering in traumatized patients: namely, that suffering makes it possible to silence an extreme pain. This is not a simple unease, but something terrifying. As Bromberg (2013) argues, trauma destabilizes the sense of self through a tsunami of chaotic affective states that the mind is unable to process. The "shadow of the tsunami" continues to torment the person, robbing them of both present and future, especially when the origin of the trauma lies in the early phases of development.

In the traumatized person's unconscious dynamics, this pain takes on the features of a spectral presence: not the Freudian *uncanny*, linked to a repressed conflict between desire and prohibition, but a primitive terror, bearer of a disorganizing and nameless anguish. Traumatophilic behaviours thus assume the function of survival-oriented defences: inflicting suffering on oneself or on the other in order to silence a traumatic pain (a spectral terror, a *Terrifying* [1]) that persists as bodily memory.

Traumatic identification helps to keep the subject psychically anchored to a past that incessantly reappears in the present in the form of repetition, both psychic and bodily. In these individuals, life choices, expectations and affective experience are guided not by desire, but by the necessity of preventing danger and containing a primary anxiety. In this sense, traumatic identification often constitutes the invisible nucleus around which compulsive behaviours, addictions, and dysfunctional relational patterns are organized: what is repeated is the relational, affective, and defensive configuration that made survival possible.

Clinically, the task is not to unmask or interpret the identification directly, but rather to co-create an *intersubjective space* within which the therapeutic dyad can continually experience itself on multiple levels – unconscious and conscious, bodily and psychic, affective and cognitive. Within this space, through an intense intertwining of feelings, fantasies, thoughts, motivations, memories, and recollections, a process of disidentification can progressively be set in motion, enabling the patient to access a freer, more flexible, and more integrated relationship with themselves and with others.

Note

1 In psychoanalytic terms, *the Uncanny* (*Das Unheimliche*; Freud, 1919) refers to a disturbing affective experience that arises from the return of what was once familiar and subsequently *repressed*, rather than from the unknown per se. It is linked to phantasmatic material that has already been symbolized and integrated into the psychic economy, and that returns in an altered, ambiguous form. The Uncanny unsettles the subject by occupying a liminal space between the familiar and the alien, preserving a fragile yet meaningful relation to the thinkable.

By contrast, *the Terrifying* designates a more radical psychic experience, grounded not in repression but in dissociation. It emerges from the irruption of what has never been symbolized and is associated with unmentalized, early relational trauma. Rather than evoking interpretative hesitation, the Terrifying activates primitive survival responses and reflects the presence of an *unrepressed* unconscious spectral figure – an unrepresented traumatic residue that inhabits the body and the relational field, remaining outside narrative and symbolic integration.

Chapter 8

Dissociative Trauma, Affect Dysregulation, and Addiction

What has been set out so far allows for a more precise clarification of what I mean when I describe addictions as a disorder linked to dissociative trauma. I would like to return to one aspect already addressed in previous chapters: namely, that addictive behaviours cannot be reduced to a simple pursuit of pleasure, nor interpreted solely as deficits of self-control or as self-destructive choices. Rather, they function as a refuge, as an "escape when there is no escape" (Putnam, 1997), enacted to ensure bodily and psychic survival when inner experience becomes excessive, unmanageable, and disorganizing. The traumatized person does not take refuge in addiction to flee a vaguely defined distress, but to withdraw from a radical, primitive pain that bears the unconscious characteristics of the *Terrifying*: an overflowing and unconscious affective experience (here the reference is to the unrepressed unconscious; Craparo, 2018; Craparo & Mucci, 2016) that does not merely unsettle, but overwhelms – threatening the continuity of the self – and cannot be represented or thought. In the presence of this pain, the body–mind is forced to find an immediate way out: a mode of sensory and mental withdrawal that interrupts contact with internal states experienced as potentially annihilating.

Addiction is therefore configured in relation to a dissociative retreat: a way of creating a protective distance from bodily memories of violent, traumatic (unmentalized) sensations and emotions that continue to be reactivated in the present (Figure 8.1).

The addictive-object makes it possible to modulate (albeit dysfunctionally) a nervous system that is constantly on alert, anaesthetizing the load of unmentalized pain (the *internal Terrifying*) stored in the body–mind's memory.

Clinical Vignettes

Mario is twenty-six and comes to therapy for a gambling addiction, which he describes as "the only way to switch off my brain". Raised by an unpredictable and violent father, he recounts a childhood constantly marked by alertness: the anguished waiting for his father to return home drunk, the fear that he might beat him and his mother, and the impossibility of feeling safe even

DOI: 10.4324/9781003325314-9

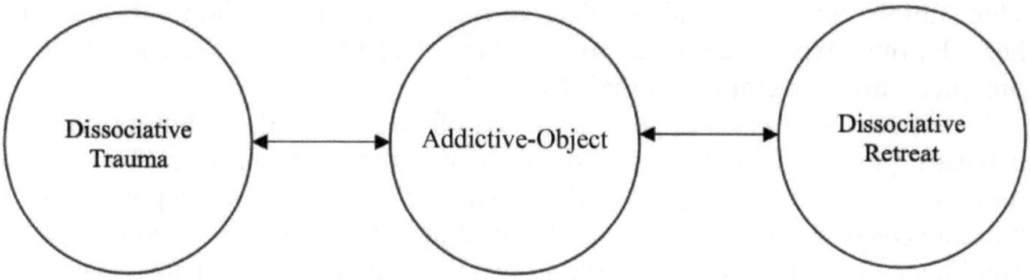

Figure 8.1 Dissociative trauma exerts a constant pressure on the body–mind system. The addictive-object acts as a means of modulation, producing a dissociative retreat that allows a temporary distance from traumatic affective states.

within the domestic space. His childhood experience appears organized around a chronic threat that was never fully mentalizable and that has profoundly shaped the regulation of his nervous system.

As an adult, Mario lives in a near-permanent state of hypervigilance. Sudden noises, relational demands or minor conflicts produce a rapid somatic escalation: tachycardia, muscular tension, shortness of breath. He does not speak of fear, nor does he recognize it as such; yet his body tells a different story. It is as though he lives constantly with the need to keep everything under control, for fear that "something frightening and incomprehensible might happen" – as he repeatedly puts it. The threat is undefined, but omnipresent, inscribed in bodily memory more than in thought.

Gambling enters the scene each evening as a addictive-object: not for pleasure, but for its anaesthetic function. In describing it, Mario uses strongly relational language, almost personifying the object: "The roulette lights take me into their arms, and then they crush me and won't let me go." Each evening, after the first bets, he experiences a sensation of slowing down, as though an internal, deafening and terrifying noise suddenly diminishes. It is at that point that he can finally not feel "assailed by a trembling that is inside – inside the muscles, inside the brain".

The effect of gambling is not euphoric, but profoundly dissociative: a muffled space, devoid of tension, in which the trembling is no longer felt. The dissociative retreat produced by gambling provides a *temporary* distance from the traumatic bodily memories that keep his nervous system in a constant state of alert. However, this loosening does not correspond to a ventral-vagal regulation grounded in safety and connection, but rather to a dorsal-vagal response of immobilization and shutdown. When the effect of gambling fades, hyperactivation returns in an amplified form, reactivating the addiction–dissociation–alertness cycle and reinforcing the compulsive need to resort once again to the object.

Sara is twenty-nine and presents with a cocaine addiction that alternates with long periods of withdrawal, immobility, and shutdown. Her developmental history is marked by profound early emotional neglect and by a cold, silent family climate devoid of affective resonance. From childhood onwards, her relational experience seems to have been shaped more by absence than by presence, more by emptiness than by conflict.

In sessions, Sara often appears switched off, with a fixed, distant gaze and a collapsed posture suggestive of a dorsal-vagal immobilization state. Her voice is monotone, movements reduced, affect scarcely accessible. She reports feeling "disconnected from my body" and spending entire days in a condition of numbness, as though she were "behind glass" – present, yet not truly participating in experience. Her suffering is not expressed through agitation, but through a sense of emptiness and absence, in which feeling itself seems suspended.

In this case, dissociative trauma does not lead to hyperactivation states, but to a predominantly hypoactive mode of functioning organized around collapse and withdrawal. Cocaine, in this context, serves a function opposite to that observable in hyperactivated clinical pictures: it does not slow or switch off, but acts as a stimulant. After using, Sara reports that she "feels alive again". In her language, feeling alive does not coincide with a shareable emotional experience, but with the perception of a body that finally reactivates, emerging from an internal sense of deadness through an intense adrenergic excitation (sympathetic system).

Here too, the substance's effect can be read as a dissociative retreat. Dissociation does not serve to reduce excessive activation, but to allow a temporary exit from collapse without coming into contact with the underlying traumatic emotions. The body is modulated from the outside – artificially reactivated – in order to avoid a direct encounter with the pain, emptiness, and despair linked to the early experience of affective non-existence. In this sense, the substance functions as a substitute autonomic regulator, allowing Sara to "feel alive" without having to feel.

Luca, forty-five, does not use substances, but presents with an addiction to online gambling and pornography. Raised within a traumatic attachment context, with an intrusive mother and an emotionally absent father, Luca learned early that relationship is a source of confusion and threat. Any request for real intimacy activates in him a sense of invasion and a disorienting experience of anguish.

The addictive-object, in this case, is not a substance but a behaviour that serves the same function as a substance: gambling and pornography create a highly structured, predictable, and controllable dissociative withdrawal. Luca describes these moments as "a place where nobody asks anything of me and I don't have to feel anything". The effect is a dissociative retreat that removes him from traumatic affective states linked to relationship, while leaving the internal fracture intact. Here too, the means does not heal the trauma, but temporarily modulates its pressure.

I would now like to propose the case of Giuliano, a sex addict whom I have already presented and discussed in a 2014 article. Although not yet included in DSM or ICD diagnostic manuals, clinical experience and research highlight features in sexual addiction that are common to other forms of addiction. According to Aviel Goodman (1998), the key characteristics that distinguish sexual addiction from other modes of sexual behaviour are essentially two: first, the individual is unable reliably to control sexual behaviour; second, the behaviour entails significantly harmful consequences and persists despite these consequences. But let us return to the clinical case.

Giuliano comes to therapy in adulthood (in reality at the insistent request of his fiancée, who was by then prepared to end their relationship unless he began psychotherapy) for compulsive sexual behaviours that he describes as increasingly intrusive and beyond his control. These behaviours include the repetitive pursuit of anonymous sexual encounters, compulsive use of pornography, and masturbation experienced as coercive, often prolonged for hours. What led him to seek help was not so much the act itself as the profound feelings of shame, emptiness, and fragmentation, accompanied by the sense of "disappearing" from himself. Giuliano reports that, in the moments immediately preceding the sexual enactment, he experiences a state of mounting internal tension, difficult to define, that he cannot translate into words and that he feels bodily as a sudden excitation, chest pressure, and an indistinct sense of urgency, accompanied by mental confusion.

His developmental history is marked by an emotionally neglectful family context. His parents are described as materially very present, but emotionally unavailable, with little capacity to recognize and mirror his emotional experience. Giuliano thus grows up without developing a shared affective language, learning early to rely on dysfunctional self-regulatory strategies. He has difficulty regulating negative emotions, especially shame, anger, and anxiety. In this scenario, compulsive sexuality intervenes as a dissociative means, as a addictive-object capable of modulating from the outside an overloaded nervous system.

The effect of this modulation is a dissociative retreat: Giuliano temporarily withdraws from the affective field, from relationship and from his sense of self, finding a momentary distance from emotional states experienced as unbearable. Yet once the effect ends after orgasm, the retreat rapidly reverses and shame, guilt, self-devaluation, and a renewed sense of fragmentation emerge, further fuelling the compulsive circuit. In this cycle, craving – as in other forms of addiction – is the expression of an obsessive–impulsive–compulsive spectrum grounded in dissociative mechanisms, aimed at preventing the emergence of unmentalized traumatic emotions.

As with other types of addiction, sexual addiction is experienced as a strategy of somato-psychic survival, rooted in a developmental trauma that has compromised the development of affect regulation and the self's reflective function.

Dissociations

The construct of dissociative trauma, as I clarified in the previous chapter, considers dissociation not as a simple effect of trauma, but as a condition immanent to its very definition: trauma, etymologically, means a wound, involving both body and psyche. In traumatized patients, this wound inscribes itself in the self as an internal fracture, giving rise to a structurally dissociated personality, which may be articulated into two or more parts.

At this point, it becomes necessary to specify the distinction between dissociation understood as a psychic mechanism, structural dissociation, and dissociative symptoms – terms that in the literature and in clinical practice are frequently used interchangeably, generating no small amount of conceptual ambiguity.

Structural Dissociation, Dissociation, and Dissociative Symptoms

To understand what is meant by this expression, we must begin with the fundamental contribution of Pierre Janet (1889) and his theory of disaggregation (*désagrégation*). Contrary to the defensive hypothesis proposed by Freud (1895), Janet held that dissociation involved a disconnection of the normally overlapping and integrated levels of mental functions due to a structural breakdown induced by violent emotions (defined by Janet as "vehement emotions") elicited by traumatic experiences. This compromise results in insufficient integration between two or more "systems of ideas and functions that constitute personality" (Janet, 1907, p. 332). These systems are not mere sets of isolated functions, but always include a sense of self, more or less developed, endowed with a first-person perspective (van der Hart & Dorahy, 2009).

Janet also observed that the disaggregation of personality was frequently accompanied by dissociative symptoms, including sensorimotor phenomena such as bodily anaesthesias or perceptual alterations (van der Hart & Dorahy, 2009; Nijenhuis, 2014). More precisely, Janet described the integrative impairment through two main processes: on the one hand, a narrowing of the field of personal consciousness; on the other, a tendency towards the separation and emancipation of the systems of ideas and functions that constitute the personality (Janet, 1907; 1909). In such a condition, the vehement emotions linked to trauma tend to replace adaptive integrative action, assuming a dominant role in psychic functioning.

Over time, however, some authors' clinical and theoretical attention has progressively shifted from dissociative personality structures to so-called dissociative responses, generating a certain conceptual confusion both about the meaning of dissociation itself and about its relationship with traumatic experiences. For example, Meares and Barral (2019) proposed distinguishing disaggregation, understood as a global disintegration of personality, from dissociation, which would refer instead to specific psychic phenomena, such as a traumatic memory that acquires a relative autonomy from the rest of mental functioning. According to these authors, the two terms should not be treated as synonymous.

Farina and colleagues (2019), while not using the term disaggregation, similarly distinguish disintegration, which manifests for example in depersonalization and derealization, from dissociation understood as an integrative failure followed by a reorganization of the personality's constituent elements into more separate forms.

In recent years, van der Hart, Nijenhuis and Steele (2006) – more aligned with Janet's thinking – have offered a rigorous theoretical systematization through their Theory of Structural Dissociation of the Personality, with the explicit aim of carrying out a "conceptual clean-up" by distinguishing structural dissociation from dissociative mechanisms and from dissociative symptoms.

According to this theory, structural dissociation involves the division of the personality into dissociative parts endowed with different functions and perspectives. Two fundamental types of parts are distinguished (van der Hart et al., 2006): the Apparently Normal Part of the Personality (ANP), oriented towards everyday functioning and avoidance of traumatic memories, and the Emotional Part of the Personality (EP), fixated at the time of trauma, which chronically relives traumatic experiences and enacts defensive survival responses (attack, flight, freezing, collapse).

The presence of a single ANP and a single EP constitutes primary structural dissociation, typical of simple post-traumatic disorders, including PTSD. In the presence of chronic or repeated trauma – especially during development, when integrative capacity is physiologically more fragile – dissociation tends to become more complex: secondary structural dissociation. In this case, a single ANP remains, but multiple EPs are present, often organized around different defensive systems or around painful affective states such as shame, loneliness, or terror. This configuration is frequent in complex PTSD, borderline personality disorder, and DDNOS subtype 1b. Tertiary structural dissociation, finally, entails the presence of multiple ANPs and multiple EPs and is characteristic of dissociative identity disorder (DID).

The model proposed by van der Hart, Nijenhuis and Steele may be understood as a neo-Janetian theory that takes up Janet's original insight regarding the link between trauma and dissociation, integrating it with contributions from affective neuroscience and contemporary psychotraumatology.

These authors stress the need not to interpret automatically symptoms characterized by a loss of information as dissociative symptoms. The discriminating criterion for speaking of dissociative symptoms is, they argue, that the subject presents a structural dissociation characterized by alternation between personality parts (EP and ANP). To give an example, forgetting a stressful event does not in itself constitute an indicator of dissociation unless it is associated with the activation of dissociative personality parts. In subjects who do not present a dissociated personality structure, a narrowing of the field of consciousness can explain forgetting without recourse to the concept of dissociation or to interpretation in terms of dissociative symptoms. This is a position not shared by everyone, particularly those who propose a broad conceptualization of dissociation, such as Bromberg (2006), for whom:

> To reiterate, dissociation is not only a mental process but also a mental structure that exists in everyone – for some people more extensively than for others – a structure that hypnoidally sequesters certain self-states and limits their communication with one another as a proactive defence against the repetition of what has already happened. This proactive defence operates when massive trauma has occurred but operates equally and in some ways even more extensively when early 'developmental trauma' has created areas of dissociative mental structure with or without subsequent massive trauma. The reason that developmental trauma (also termed relational trauma) is of such significance is that it shapes the attachment patterns that establish what is to become a stable or unstable core self. [...]
>
> Dissociation is a defence unlike any other. It protects the stability of the self by controlling unsymbolized traumatic affect that it cannot regulate. It is not simply a different term for the concept of repression. Repression defines a process that is designed to avoid disavowed mental content that may lead to unpleasant intrapsychic conflict. Dissociation shows its signature not by disavowing aspects of mental *contents* per se, but through the patient's alienation from aspects of *self* that are inconsistent with his experience of 'me' at a given moment. It functions because conflict is *unbearable* to the mind, not because it is *unpleasant*
>
> (pp.6–7; italics in the original).

Considering identity as a multiplicity of mental states, dissociation does not necessarily represent a pathological condition for Bromberg.

> What was formerly normal dissociation, the loose configuration of multiple self-states that enables a person to 'feel like one self while being many,' becomes rigidified into a dissociative mental structure (the most extreme form of which we know as 'multiple personality' or 'dissociative identity disorder'), each self now uncompromisingly boundaried within its specific pattern of interpersonal engagement that gives its self-meaning the cast of truth. Because the individual states are defensively and rigidly isolated from one another, the dissociative structure has not only been restored but now is able to protect indefinitely the subjective sense of self-consistency and continuity by locating personal identity tightly within whichever self-state has access to consciousness and cognition at a given moment. The security of the personality is now linked to a trauma-based view of reality whereby the person is always ready for the disaster that he is sure is around the next corner, and some dissociated aspect of self is 'on-call' to deal with it. The price that is paid is that the individual can no longer afford to feel safe even when he is
>
> (1998/2001, pp. 12–13).

Unlike non-pathological dissociative conditions, dissociative disorders express a pathological dissociation between disaggregated and non-communicating self-states, in which the individual loses the capacity to 'stand in the spaces' – to move creatively from one state to another and to respond adaptively to environmental demands.

This is, as noted, a broad conceptualization of dissociation, not aligned with Janet's original formulation. Unlike Janet's theory, Bromberg emphasizes the intersubjective and processual dimension of dissociation, highlighting its communicative function within the therapeutic relationship, in the condition known as enactment. Bromberg writes:

> Through enactment, the dissociated affective experience is communicated from within a shared 'not-me' cocoon (Bromberg, 1998) until it is cognitively and linguistically symbolized through relational negotiation. In the early phase of an enactment, the shared dissociative cocoon supports implicit communication without mental representation. Within this cocoon, when the patient's self-state that is organizing the immediate relationship switches, the therapist's self-state also switches, equally dissociatively, to a state that over time can receive and react to the patient's dissociated state-switch
>
> (2008, p. 337).

In this passage, Bromberg highlights how enactment does not merely represent a failure of mentalization but constitutes a transitional mode of communication when symbolic functioning is temporarily unavailable. Within the shared dissociative cocoon, both participants become involved in an intersubjective field in which affect is conveyed implicitly, through bodily states, shifts in attention, and variations in emotional tone, rather than through reflective thought. It is crucial to emphasize that the therapist's participation in this field does not imply a collapse of therapeutic function nor a symmetrical dissociation, but rather takes the form of a controlled and reversible involvement that preserves reflective capacity. It is precisely this possibility of remaining partially within the enactment while simultaneously maintaining a reflective stance that enables the therapist, over time, to metabolize dissociated affect and to facilitate its gradual transformation into experience that can be thought about, named, and symbolized. From this perspective, enactment emerges as a necessary phase of the therapeutic process, allowing dissociated self-states to enter the relational field before they can be integrated into a meaningful narrative.

Conclusion

On the basis of what has been set out, I propose that the construct of dissociation may be articulated in two principal senses: (1) as a structural condition of the personality, characterized by a division into relatively autonomous parts; and (2) as an active and unconscious defensive mechanism.

With regard to structural dissociation, understood as the outcome of a rupture in the unity of personality sustained by traumatic emotional states, it is possible to distinguish three terms frequently used in the literature as synonyms: disaggregation, disgregation, and disintegration. In *Theory and Clinical Practice of Dissociative Trauma* (2026), I proposed considering disaggregation and *fragmentation* as essentially equivalent concepts, insofar as they describe a splitting of mental functioning into parts, as observed for example in borderline personality disorder, dissociative identity disorder, and post-traumatic stress disorder; the term disintegration, by contrast, refers to a deeper and more complex rupture of the unity of the self (a *shattering*), found in psychosis.

The term dissociation does not necessarily imply the presence of disaggregation or disintegration of the personality, but may also be configured as a psychic defence to which the individual resorts in order to distance themselves from excessively intense affective states, without this necessarily entailing a structural fracture of the self. Structural dissociation and defensive dissociation therefore represent two different forms of dissociation and should not be confused.

With regard to dissociative symptoms, in line with van der Hart, Nijenhuis and Steele (2006), I maintain that symptoms may properly be considered dissociative only when they are connected to an underlying structural dissociative condition.

A similar line of reasoning can also be applied to addictions. It is indeed possible to observe a repeated use of a addictive-object without this necessarily implying the presence of an addiction disorder. In order to formulate a diagnosis of addiction, it is necessary to diagnose a structural dissociation of the self, a condition typical of dissociative trauma disorders. From this perspective, the frequent alterations of consciousness, perception, memory, and identity observable in addicted patients may be understood as dissociative symptoms – expressions of a psychic organization founded on the division of the self and on the difficulty of integrating experience.

It is within this framework that I understand addiction as the expression of a reactivation of traumatic memories lodged in one or more dissociative parts of the personality, which drives the subject to resort to counterphobic strategies through the use of addictive-objects, understood as modes of self-medication oriented towards survival (Figure 8.2).

In Figure 8.2 I have included additional elements, compared with Figure 8.1, that allow for a more articulated understanding of addictions. As emerges from the diagram – to be read clockwise, starting from traumatic memories – biological, psychological, and social variables intervene at every stage of the addictive process: from the activation of traumatic memories, through addiction memory, to the dissociative refuge elicited by

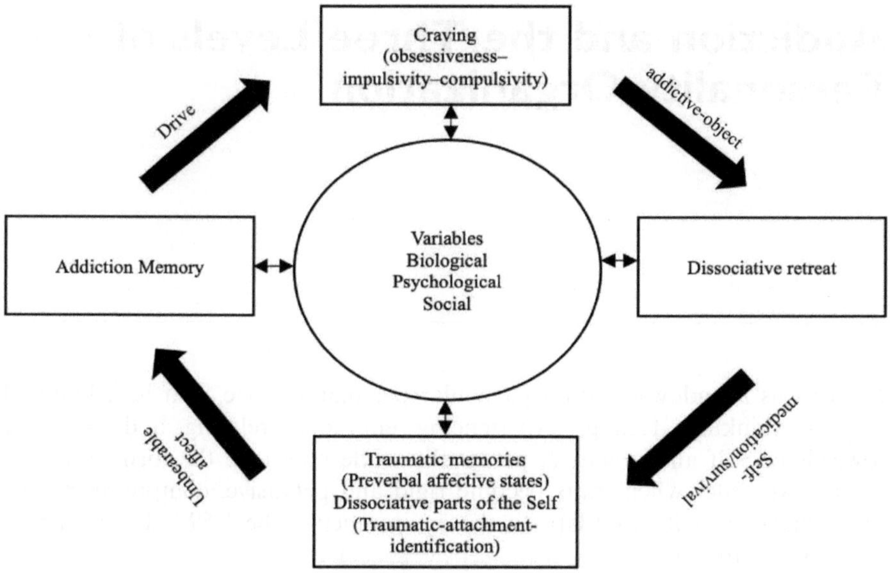

Figure 8.2 Dimensions of the addictive process

the addictive-object. This model leads us to conceptualize addictions as expressions of affect dysregulation, what Khantzian (1985) has described in terms of a *self-regulation disorder*: behaviours that provide an apparently regulatory, yet in reality dysfunctional, support to painful affective states, thereby maintaining the addictive cycle and reinforcing traumatic experience.

Chapter 9

Addiction and the Three Levels of Personality Organization

Each of us is endowed with a particular personality style, that is, a habitual way of thinking, feeling, experiencing emotions, relating and behaving towards oneself and others. A personality style may take the form of a personality disorder when traits become rigid and pervasive, compromising the individual's capacity to adapt to the environment. The DSM defines a personality disorder as

> an enduring pattern of inner experience and behaviour that deviates markedly from the expectations of the individual's culture, is pervasive and inflexible, has an onset in adolescence or early adulthood, is stable over time, and leads to distress or impairment
>
> (APA, 2013, p. 645).

In psychoanalysis, personality is assessed along a continuum ranging from healthy mental functioning to psychotic functioning, passing through neurotic and borderline functioning. These are referred to as levels of personality organization, within which specific mental disorders – including addictions – are located.

The aim of this chapter is to bring into dialogue two ways of understanding the patient that, although operating on different levels, are profoundly interconnected: descriptive psychiatric diagnosis and psychodynamically informed structural diagnosis. In clinical work, indeed, the classification of symptoms does not exhaust the need to understand how a person organizes their inner experience, relationships, and affects.

Among the contributions that have most successfully attempted to bridge this gap, Otto Kernberg's proposal (1975; 1984) deserves particular recognition for translating the complexity of structural diagnosis into an observable and clinically usable system, articulating personality functioning along seven fundamental dimensions. From this perspective, personality organizations are not conceived as rigid labels, but as relatively stable configurations of psychic functioning that orient the way in which the subject perceives themselves, others, and reality.

DOI: 10.4324/9781003325314-10

The neurotic, borderline, and psychotic levels of personality organization (Table 9.1) thus represent different modes of psychic containment in the face of conflicts, affects, and relational demands. Their main characteristics, as they emerge in clinical practice, are summarized below.

1 Identity

Identity refers both to the organization and to the contents of the subject's internal world. An integrated and relatively stable internal experience of self and other underpins the subjective sense of self-cohesion and is associated with behavioural correlates such as the capacity to invest in work and to build intimate and enduring relationships. By contrast, a non-integrated sense of self and other is associated with a fragmentation (borderline level) or a shattering (psychotic level) of identity.

Table 9.1 The three clinically relevant levels of personality organization

	Neurotic	*Borderline*	*Psychotic*
Identity	Integrated (in some cases, the sense of self and others may be moderately superficial)	Mild to moderate impairment of identity	Diffuse
Object relations	Stable, complex (may show some difficulty with empathy or in integrating tenderness and eroticism)	Unstable, superficial, short-lived; may be controlling in order to avoid abandonment anxiety	Absence of stable, intimate relationships
Defensive levels	Mature defences (some individuals may make rare use of primitive defences)	Immature / primitive defences	Immature / primitive defences
Reality testing	Intact; may show perceptual distortions (mild–moderate)	Characterized by moderate to severe perceptual distortions associated with dissociative processes	Not intact, with severe perceptual distortions
Coping	Moderately or severely rigid (and vulnerable to stress)	Maladaptive	Maladaptive
Aggression	Mild to moderate difficulties in aggression	Primitive aggression; difficulties in managing aggression, especially self-directed; in more severe forms also other-directed	Primitive and poorly modulated, especially under conditions of stress
Moral values	Inflexible or rigid and vulnerable to stress	Variable; in some cases poorly integrated	Severely non-integrated

2 Object Relations

This dimension concerns both the quality of the subject's interpersonal relationships and the nature of the internal experience of self and other. At the intrapsychic level, the quality of object relations is defined by the degree of integration, stability, and depth of internal representations, as well as by the capacity for affective investment in significant relationships.

3 Defence Mechanisms

Defence mechanisms are largely unconscious and serve to protect the individual from emotional stress and internal conflict. A distinction is made between primary defences, typical of earlier developmental phases and of more archaic psychic functioning – such as splitting, idealization and devaluation, primitive denial, projective identification, somatization, and recourse to fantasy – and secondary defences, which are more mature and characteristic of higher-level functioning, such as intellectualization, rationalization, repression, moralization, and more adaptive forms such as humour.

4 Reality Testing

This refers to the capacity to distinguish between stimuli of internal and external origin, as well as to evaluate one's own intrapersonal and interpersonal functioning in relation to socially shared criteria of reality. Intact reality testing allows for flexible and coherent adaptation to the external world, whereas its impairment signals more severe levels of personality disorganization.

5 Coping/Rigidity

This dimension concerns the individual's capacity to respond flexibly and adaptively to potentially stressful situations, reducing emotional distress and dealing constructively with environmental demands. Rigidity, by contrast, indicates a chronic tendency to react in automatic and stereotyped ways that are poorly adaptive.

6 Aggression

The quality of aggression refers to the degree to which the subject's inner life and behaviour are dominated by aggressive impulses and by the defences mobilized to control them. It is assessed through the presence of destructive or self-destructive behaviours, sadism, an omnipotent control of others, and feelings of hatred. A predominance of aggression is generally associated with the use of primitive defences and with poor-quality object relations.

7 Moral Values

This dimension concerns the degree of internalization of moral values and norms capable of influencing the subject's inner experience and orienting behaviour. Morality is assessed through modes of ethical decision-making and the capacity to experience guilt in relation to one's actions.

Individuals with a borderline personality organization present a structurally dissociated identity, reflected in unstable interpersonal relationships and marked affective lability. Affective states tend to oscillate rapidly between opposite poles, shifting from intensely negative experiences to moments of apparent wellbeing and back again. This is associated with a variable – though often significant – impairment in mentalization capacity. The defence mechanisms predominantly employed are of a primary type, in particular splitting, projective identification, idealization/devaluation, denial, and dissociation. As long as stressful stimuli are not activated, reality testing may appear substantially adequate; however, this is only an apparent normality, since the underlying personality structure remains fragile and dissociated. Under conditions of emotional stress, the perception of reality becomes mildly to moderately distorted, coping strategies prove rigid and maladaptive, and forms of primitive, poorly modulated aggression emerge.

In psychotic personality organizations, by contrast, a traumatic disintegration of identity is observed. The boundaries between self and other, reality and fantasy, inner and outer world are profoundly compromised, making it extremely difficult to construct and maintain a stable and coherent sense of self. In response to emotional stress, the mind resorts to archaic and ineffective defence mechanisms (delusional projection, psychotic denial, psychotic distortion) in an attempt to contain persecutory anxiety and fears of collapse. Reality testing appears severely impaired, as evidenced by hallucinations, delusional ideation, and profoundly disorganized thinking, rendering contact with external reality fragile, intermittent, and often incomprehensible to the relational environment.

In neurotic personality organizations, identity appears globally integrated, and the boundaries between self and other, as well as between inner and outer reality, are largely preserved. The subject maintains adequate reality testing and continuity of the sense of self, although unresolved intrapsychic conflicts and repressed contents may generate symptoms, suffering, and character rigidity. In the face of emotional stress, the mind predominantly resorts to more evolved defence mechanisms – such as repression, displacement, rationalization, intellectualization, denial, isolation of affect, undoing, and reaction formation – which, although sometimes costly in terms of symptom formation, allow for a relative stability of psychic and relational functioning. Anxiety is predominantly conflictual and symbolizable, linked to desire, guilt, and loss, and can be mentalized and represented within a coherent narrative framework.

In a recent study conducted on a group of 30 participants with a confirmed diagnosis of severe addiction, formulated according to DSM-5 criteria and predominantly related to cocaine use, we assessed the level of personality organization using the STIPO.[1] The results showed that none of the participants exhibited neurotic mental functioning: the majority (22 participants) fell within a borderline personality organization, while the remainder presented a psychotic organization.

In all of these individuals, addictive symptoms were closely linked to the reactivation of traumatic memories and to the emergence of unmentalized affective states.

In my clinical experience, by contrast with patients with borderline and psychotic personality organizations, in patients with a neurotic personality organization the use of a addictive-object appears more frequently attributable to unconscious conflicts and symbolic dynamics. This distinction has important psychotherapeutic implications: at the borderline and psychotic levels, treatment should be oriented primarily towards affect regulation, the stabilization of psychic functioning, and the construction of a sense of safety; in the case of a neurotic organization, therapeutic intervention can instead focus on interpretative work and the elaboration of unconscious conflicts.

Addictive Symptoms and Structural Diagnosis

If there is one merit that can be attributed to psychoanalysis, it is that it does not conceive of the symptom reductively as a mere 'malfunction' that obstructs the individual's wellbeing and should therefore be eliminated as quickly as possible, but rather as a phenomenon that must be questioned in order to understand its nature, its unconscious implications, its relationship to personality structure, and the possible transformative developments it contains.

Following Freud's intuition, the symptom represents an authentic response to a form of suffering that is far more complex than it appears on the surface. It is within this perspective that the distinction I proposed (Craparo, 2008) between *symptom-as-sign* and *symptom-as-symbol* acquires meaning: the former indicates the presence of developmental deficits in mentalization and affect regulation; the latter refers instead to repressed and interpretable conflicts.

The Symptom in Psychotic Personality Organizations

In psychotic organizations, the symptom takes the form of a symptom-as-sign. In these cases, the psychic structure lacks the tools necessary to transform inner experience into representations endowed with symbolic–verbal meaning; consequently, the symptom emerges as an immediate manifestation of a failure in processes of psychic integration. It is in these terms that delusions and hallucinations may be understood: not as expressions of repressed conflict, but as primitive affective states that have not yet encountered a mental container capable of elaborating them symbolically. In these configurations, the symptom does not speak – it signals. And what it signals is precisely a structural limit in the capacity to regulate and represent emotional experience.

The Symptom in Borderline Personality Organizations

Within borderline organization, a distinction is made between low-functioning and high-functioning levels. In low-functioning borderline organization – closer to psychosis – the symptom assumes characteristics very similar to those observed in psychotic structures. In these cases, however, there is no true shattering of the personality – as in full-blown psychoses – but rather a *fragmentation* that preserves some intact nuclei of self-functioning within an overall profoundly unstable framework. The capacity for symbolization is severely compromised, affects are difficult to regulate, and the symptom emerges as a direct signal of deficit rather than as the expression of a representable conflict.

There is a difference with high-functioning borderline organizations, in which the symptom displays a more hybrid nature. Although it lacks the stability and coherence found in neurotic organizations, the symptom may contain a rudimentary symbolic meaning. The capacity to represent inner states is present but fragile: some emotional experiences can be translated into symbolic forms, while others still collapse into more primitive signalling modes. This results in a continuous oscillation between moments of understanding and moments of loss of integration, making the symptom a site in which residues of deficit coexist with attempts at symbolization.

The Symptom in Neurotic Personality Organizations

When personality structure is intact, as in neurosis, the symptom takes on fully symbolic characteristics, that is, it functions as a compromise formation that allows the psyche to express repressed conflicts through a metaphorical language. Here, although the symptom is a source of distress, it possesses an internal (unconscious) logic and is therefore interpretable, insofar as it pertains to an unconscious structured like a language (the repressed unconscious) and is endowed with representations and associative links. In these cases, the symptom not only speaks, but can be translated, rendered thinkable, and transformed over the course of analytic work.

Addictive Symptoms in Relation to the Three Levels of Personality Organization

In my view, the notion of the addictive symptom acquires its full meaning when it is considered in relation to the three levels of personality organization. It does not represent a symptomatic form autonomous from the symptom-as-sign or the symptom-as-symbol, but rather a particular modality that the symptom may assume depending on the integrative capacities of the psychic apparatus. In psychotic organizations, as well as in borderline organizations (both low- and high-functioning), the addictive symptom is not merely the manifestation of a deficit in symbolization: it contains, anaesthetizes, or wards off internal tensions that would otherwise be unbearable. These are somato-psychic refuges through which the subject desperately attempts to maintain continuity of the self or to avoid the fear of identity collapse (the latter being particularly relevant in psychosis), in contexts where symbolic functions are insufficiently developed – or entirely lacking – to fulfil this task.

In neurotic organizations, by contrast, when the symptom appears it represents the specific expression of an unconscious conflict. In this case we are dealing with symptoms of a symbolic–verbal nature, metaphors of the unsayable – unsayable because they have been repressed. In psychoanalytic terms, the neurotic symptom is sustained by an unconscious phantasy (repressed – the so-called *Uncanny*), whereas in borderline and psychotic patients the symptom is related to an unconscious spectre (unrepressed and dissociated), which I have termed the *Terrifying*.

It is enough to listen to a neurotic patient to grasp an existence regulated by an internal motto shaped by duty, control, and adherence to internalized rules, often accompanied by a marked sense of guilt and a constant conflict between desire and prohibition: *I would like to, but I cannot because I must*. This is characteristic of the neurotic patient, devoted to the renunciation (*I cannot*) of their desires (*I would like to*) in order to comply with an internalized super-egoic/sabotaging demand (*because I must*), the result of the internalization of particularly rigid family relationship patterns. These figures recall the necessity of sacrifice and threaten guilt and punishment should the individual allow space for their own personal and emotional inclinations, their desires – in other words, should they decide to 'be and become' themselves in accordance with their emotional truth. The neurotic patient lives within an (learned) impotence with which they have identified and from which they are unable to free themselves. This impotence is embodied (in some cases taking the form of male or female sexual difficulties, such as premature ejaculation, erectile failure, anorgasmia, vaginismus etc.) and translates into a loss of emotional authenticity. Neurotic symptomatology thus refers to a message to be deciphered, originating in an internal conflict between fear and curiosity, between what is permitted (complying with duty) and what is desired but forbidden (accessing one's own desire), between duty and freedom. This conflict is most often resolved through recourse to mature (secondary) defences, such as repression, intellectualization, moralization, and denial, along with behaviours associated with these mechanisms.

In these patients, the use of a addictive-object does not respond to the need to preserve functional capacity, but rather to silence repressed contents that disturb psychophysical equilibrium. Such individuals may develop forms of dependence in the absence of craving; for this reason, rather than addiction in the strict sense, it may be more appropriate to speak of a dependent relationship embedded within a mental functioning characterized by rigid personality traits and a low propensity for change. This resistance is in fact linked to anxiety associated with contact with one's own emotions and desires, which may lead to the development of dependent modalities, both with respect to substances and at the relational level.

I therefore believe that assessing the level of personality organization allows the clinician to understand the nature of the addictive symptom in its manifestation as either sign or symbol (Figure 9.1), thereby assisting both prognostic formulation and the choice of psychotherapeutic intervention.

Figure 9.1 offers an articulated reading of dependence behaviours and addiction in relation to the three levels of personality organization, highlighting a progression from neurotic to psychotic functioning. From this perspective, the use of a addictive-object is not interpreted as a unitary phenomenon, but rather as a symptom that assumes different meanings and functions depending on the underlying personality structure.

In neurotic functioning, dependence behaviours are embedded within a globally integrated personality, with intact reality testing and a predominant reliance on mature defence mechanisms. In these cases, the use of the addictive-object assumes a symbolic value, expressing unconscious conflicts and repressed contents that disturb psychic equilibrium without significantly compromising the continuity of the self. Dependence, rather than addiction proper, is therefore configured in relation to this level of personality organization.

Moving along the continuum towards borderline organization, addictive behaviours become more pervasive and compulsive. The personality appears

	Neurotic	**Borderline**	**Psychotic**
Symptom type	Symptom-as-symbol	Symptom-as-sign	Symptom-as-sign
Underlying dynamics	Unconscious conflict	Traumatic memories	Traumatic memories
Defences	Mature defences	Primary defences	Primary defences
Personality organisation	Integrated personality	Disaggregated personality	Disintegrated personality
Reality testing	Intact	Mildly to moderately impaired	Severely impaired
Behavioural expression	Dependence behaviours	Addictive behaviours	Addictive behaviours

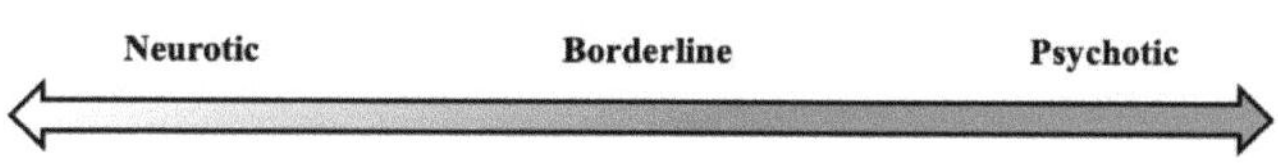

Figure 9.1 Symptomatic characteristics, dependence, addiction, and levels of personality organization

disaggregated, and reality testing is mildly to moderately compromised. Within this configuration, addiction functions as a dissociative modality oriented towards managing intense and disorganizing traumatic affects.

Finally, in psychotic organization, addiction is situated within a framework of disintegrated personality. Here, addictive behaviour is directed towards containing primitive anxieties of shattering, persecution, or annihilation. The addictive-object becomes an essential and immediate support to prevent psychic collapse.

Taken as a whole, Figure 9.1 invites us to read dependence behaviours and addiction not as isolated diagnostic entities, but as expressions of specific modes of personality functioning. Within this framework, understanding behaviour loses its purely categorical character and is situated within a dimensional and structural logic. The integration of descriptive diagnosis with the assessment of the level of personality organization thus becomes a clinically indispensable step, as it allows therapeutic choices to be oriented and interventions to be calibrated more closely to the patient's structural resources and vulnerabilities.

Note

1 The Structured Interview of Personality Organization (STIPO; Clarkin, Caligor, Stern, & Kernberg, 2007; https://www.borderlinedisorders.com/assets/Structured-Interview-of-Personality-Organization.pdf) is a semi-structured interview developed on the basis of Kernberg's structural interview, designed to assess the level of personality organization.

Chapter 10

The Monkey on One's Back

I first encountered this expression through G., who mentioned it to me during a session and suggested that I read William S. Burroughs' autobiography *Junky*, published in Italian as *La scimmia sulla schiena* (The Monkey on One's Back). The Italian title struck me immediately for its ability to condense, in a simple and powerful image, the profoundly unequal relationship between the addicted person and drugs.

This expression has long circulated within the language of addiction and is striking for its immediacy. It is a turn of phrase that belongs to those who have lived the experience of addiction from the inside, to those who know its weight not second-hand, but because they have carried it in their own flesh. Many of those who have never experienced it tend to regard it as an excessive, almost theatrical metaphor. Those who have carried it know, on the contrary, that it is an all-too-accurate description.

G. told me that at the beginning of his "career as an addict" there was no monkey. The first joints, the first lines of cocaine, were accompanied by an ecstatic sense of pleasure, relief, and encouragement.

"At the beginning it's like that for everyone," G. told me. It is a simple gesture that seems to work: a drink that lowers the noise in one's head, a dose that brings the world back into focus, a bet that makes the heart beat faster. At this stage, the addictive-object is not yet experienced as a prison, but as a solution. It's an initial source of pleasure that gradually becomes an effective way of interrupting a disturbing internal state, of silencing a tension that is difficult to name. Then the monkey arrives. The gesture ceases to be a choice and becomes a compulsion.

From a clinical standpoint, this passage marks a crucial threshold: addictive behaviour becomes organized around urgency. Use no longer responds to a conscious decision, but to a need experienced as vital. It is here that the addictive process begins to structure itself as a privileged mode of affect regulation, as self-medication, as a survival strategy.

The monkey climbs onto one's shoulders without asking permission. It does not attack, it does not openly threaten. On the contrary, it leaves the subject with the illusion of control. From time to time it climbs down, just enough to

DOI: 10.4324/9781003325314-11

allow the thought: "I can do without it." Then it climbs back up, becoming a little heavier each time. This intermittent movement is one of the most deceptive aspects of addiction: it feeds the belief that one can decide, while progressively narrowing the space of choice.

Over time, the monkey learns to know the body better than the mind. It recognizes the signals even before they become thoughts: the tremor, the sweating, the irritability, that visceral sensation that precedes every word. This is the language of craving – a preverbal, somatic language that bypasses reflection and places the will in check.

In G., the monkey had, as already mentioned, a name: Bronson. "Don't make such a fuss. You know it ends better if you give me what I want – what you want too," Bronson would tell him.

When this part appears – a part that bears the marks of a traumatic past – as happened with G., the subject gives in. Not for pleasure, but to silence a lacerating emotional pain. He thus becomes enslaved to the drug, whose use is no longer oriented towards the search for euphoria, but for anaesthesia from affective states experienced as overwhelming: a dissociative refuge that promises a temporary truce.

And so the subject learns to lie. First to others, then to himself.

- It's the last time.
- I have everything under control.
- I can stop whenever I want.

These phrases are not simple self-deceptions: they are desperate attempts to preserve an image of oneself compatible with one's history and values. The monkey knows them well. It settles comfortably on top of them, smirking.

Every addiction, although shaped in relation to its specific addictive-object (substances, alcohol, sex, and so on), follows the same grammar: urgency, promise, blackmail. Little by little, the future is mortgaged. The subject is convinced that without that object they cannot survive. This amounts to a form of procedural learning that induces the person to live in a constant state of alarm requiring disengagement responses. And given the way addiction has reorganized psychic functioning, this conviction is not entirely unfounded.

When it takes over, something dramatic happens. The body slows down, the gaze drops. One no longer walks; one drags one's feet. The monkey is no longer merely on one's back; it has become internal, part of the functioning itself. It is no longer just a behaviour, but a way of being. As Burroughs writes:

> Junk takes everything and gives nothing but insurance against junk sickness. Every now and then I took a good look at the deal I was giving myself and decided to take the cure. When you are getting plenty of junk, kicking looks easy. You say: "I'm not getting any kick from the shots anymore. I might as well quit." But when you cut down into junk sickness, the picture looks

> different. […] I knew that I did not want to go on taking junk. If I could have made a single decision, I would have decided no more junk ever. But when it came to the process of quitting, I did not have the drive. It gave me a terrible feeling of helplessness to watch myself break every schedule I set up as though I did not have control over my actions
>
> (1977, pp. 123–24).

Yet, as in G.'s case, something unexpected can sometimes occur. A tiny, almost imperceptible crack opens. A no. A fragile, trembling no to that repetition of death. To this timid no, the monkey reacts: it screams, tightens its grip, instils fear. Anxiety increases, the body aches. But for the first time, the monkey's command is not absolute.

It is then that it becomes possible to grasp an essential clinical truth: the monkey does not go away all at once. It does not fall, it does not die. It withdraws slowly – by centimetres, through attempts, through relapses. Therapeutic work consists in containing its power, in helping the person to revitalize an inner world made up of spectres – that is, internal objects that have been suffocated and whose development have been obstructed.

Each time the weight lessens, even slightly, the back hurts. Because carrying it had become a habit. But beneath this new pain something unprecedented emerges: the patient begins to feel, to feel themselves existing – I feel, therefore I am.

Along the therapeutic path, it is important to remain aware that the monkey is lying in wait, especially in the early phases of treatment, ready to climb back up. In the therapy of these patients, it is crucial that they acquire a fundamental awareness: the monkey does not coincide with the person. It is a part, a survival strategy that once had a function and that can now be transformed. It is this awareness – fragile, yet real – that makes clinical work possible and opens the way to the possibility of a life no longer organized around the compulsive use of one or more addictive-objects, but oriented towards relationship, desire, and choice.

What has been described are the stages of G.'s story – stages of a therapeutic process that unfolded over many years, seven years, marked by arduous ascents, moments of stalemate, gradual improvements, and devastating relapses. Years in which the monkey tirelessly attempted to sabotage every glimmer of hope, every impulse towards life, every possibility of change.

But they were also years in which G., not without fear, chose to place his trust in our therapeutic relationship – a relationship he slowly learned to trust and rely upon, contributing to the co-creation of an intersubjective space in which he could begin to do something new: gradually to endure emotional pain without anaesthetizing it, but by sharing it and making it thinkable for both of us. He had begun to understand that this pain was evoked by the activation of his traumatic memories – memories of toxic and violent family relationships, of interpersonal experiences that had left a deep and silent wound. A wound that, through long and patient clinical work – conducted together with other colleagues – could gradually heal, allowing him no longer to feel ashamed of himself, of his past and present life.

The therapeutic process did not erase all of G.'s vulnerabilities. It did, however, allow him to take his life back into his own hands, with a greater awareness of his limits, his vulnerabilities, and of a past that can be remembered without being relived.

Chapter 11

Treating Addiction

General Considerations

Why should a patient who already possesses their own solution – albeit a harmful and self-destructive one such as drugs – seek help from someone who will inevitably invite them to give it up? This dynamic helps to explain the often marked difficulty people with addiction experience in seeking professional help spontaneously. Indeed, it is not uncommon for the request for intervention to originate not from the patient themselves, but from external sources – family members, friends, institutions, or judicial authorities – who become aware of the consequences of addictive behaviour before the individual is able to recognize its defensive meaning and internal cost.

Fortunately, we now have a range of evidence-based treatments which, despite their different theoretical orientations, share a common underlying approach. Models such as Jan Winhall's *The Felt Sense Polyvagal Model* (2021), Felicity de Zulueta's *Traumatic Attachment Induction Procedure* (TAIP, 2025), and other related interventions are situated within a bottom-up approach, focused on bodily sensations and physiological states implicated in compulsive addictive behaviours. This methodological convergence reflects a growing clinical awareness: addicted patients do not call upon the therapist to focus exclusively on substance-use behaviours, but also – and above all – on what those behaviours are desperately attempting to help them escape from, namely internal states experienced as disorganizing and associated with unmentalized traumatic memories. From this perspective, therapeutic intervention should begin with the body's sensory experiences and physiological responses, helping the patient to transform raw and disorganized sensations into progressively more integrated mental states. This process entails a gradual translation of bodily sensations associated with addictive behaviours into sensory images (emotions) and, subsequently, into thinkable and communicable experiences (feelings). It is through this pathway – sensations–emotions–feelings – that the patient can progressively reclaim their affective experience, develop greater emotional regulation capacity, and reduce reliance on the addictive-object as the sole means of psychic survival.

Before any technical intervention, however – as clinical work itself teaches us, and as patients often indicate more or less implicitly – a fundamental

DOI: 10.4324/9781003325314-12

precondition is required, one that demands time, tact, and particular sensitivity on the part of the therapist: the construction of a sufficiently safe setting. Only when the patient begins to experience the therapeutic relationship as non-threatening does the constant state of alertness that compels them to defend themselves through addictive behaviour gradually diminish. It is within this framework that the patient can slowly develop a sense of trust and begin to rely on the therapist, experimenting with the possibility of deactivating a form of procedural learning that has contributed to a bottom-up hijacking, whereby the organism has responded automatically to threat in the absence of awareness of real danger.

Relational safety thus becomes the indispensable foundation upon which all subsequent work of affect regulation, emotional integration, and the transformation of traumatic experience – and consequently of the compulsive recourse to addictive-objects – can be built.

During one session, G. stated that through our work together he had come to understand a truth that was essential for him: our relationship had met his need to feel welcomed, understood, and recognized. That statement, simple only in appearance, encapsulated with extraordinary clarity what clinical experience and trauma research have taught me over time: *listening, understanding, compassion, participation*, and *recognition* of suffering constitute the core of truly effective therapeutic intervention with traumatized patients, including those with addiction. It is these factors that make possible – prior to any technique – the experience of relational safety, without which no transformative process can begin.

Listening lies at the heart of clinical work, but it cannot be understood as a merely cognitive activity, oriented towards quickly fitting the patient and their narrative into predefined diagnostic categories or 'manualized' responses. The listening to which I refer involves the therapist in their entirety: mind and body, cognition and emotion, conscious and unconscious. It is a form of listening that the clinician directs simultaneously towards the patient, towards themselves, and towards the therapeutic relationship – capable of grasping what is taking shape within the therapeutic field and of transforming raw, unrepresented emotions into progressively thinkable and symbolizable contents. This is an embodied form of listening, oriented towards fostering the patient's awareness of their bodily sensations – an awareness supported by a therapist who is able to listen to their own body and to the patient's body in reciprocal relation. As Winhall (2021) writes: "Listening to the bodily knowing, informed by the nervous system and our awareness, reveals our own unique direction in healing" (p. 17).

Understanding is an experience of mentalization. The word *understanding* derives from Old English *understandan*, meaning *to comprehend, grasp, or apprehend*. The verb is composed of *under* (meaning *among, between, in the midst of*) and *standan* (*to stand*). In its original sense, *to understand* did not primarily refer to a purely intellectual operation, but rather to the capacity to *stand within* or *stand among* an experience.

From a psychoanalytic perspective, understanding refers to a shared and relational process in which the therapist attunes to the patient's unconscious (unrepressed) inner world.

To feel understood means to perceive that someone is able to hold our emotional experience in mind, even if only temporarily. In early development, this experience forms the basis of secure attachment: when a child feels understood by a mentalizing caregiver, it is as though they feel themselves to exist in the caregiver's mind. In therapy, understanding takes shape as a relational stance grounded in the therapist's genuine interest in the patient's subjectivity – and vice versa. Because this is a dynamic and reciprocal process, understanding the other is inseparable from understanding oneself. Within this reciprocal exchange, understanding assumes the form of imaginative knowing, capable of making sense of one's own conscious and unconscious experiences in relation to those of the other.

Compassion represents another crucial element in work with addicted patients. It involves the therapist's capacity to attune in an emotionally authentic way to the patient's suffering. When it occurs, the experience of genuine compassion can be progressively internalized by the patient, fostering greater tolerance of their own pain. This is not a rational or voluntary effort but requires a willingness to come into emotional contact with the other's suffering, recognizing it with empathy and solidarity. In this sense, compassion – both that offered by the therapist and that which the patient gradually learns to direct towards themselves – assumes a profoundly transformative value, enabling meaning to be attributed to pain and initiating a process of symbolic elaboration of traumatic experience.

Alongside compassion, the therapist's *participation* is equally decisive. A participatory therapist is a present therapist, who adopts an active, involved, and responsive stance within the therapeutic relationship. Forms of participation may also include self-disclosure (Craparo, 2024), understood as the calibrated sharing of emotional experiences, countertransference reactions, enactments, or personal aspects, when this is functional to the therapeutic process. In whatever form it is expressed – through empathic validation, recognition, affirmation, or self-disclosure – the therapist's active participation offers the patient a concrete experience of closeness and support, facilitating the co-creation of a sufficiently secure bond.

Recognition represents one of the fundamental pillars of intersubjectivity. It entails both knowing and being known, and is manifested in those 'moments of meeting' in which the individual comes to perceive the other's genuine interest. In therapy, recognition allows the patient to feel seen as a separate subject, endowed with their own emotions, desires, and intentions. The clinical relationship thus becomes a space of co-construction in which the patient can develop greater self-awareness and acceptance of themselves and their history, opening the possibility of profound and lasting change.

All these attitudes contribute to the construction of a secure base within the therapeutic relationship: an indispensable framework within which it becomes possible to work with the body and with the psychic elaboration of traumatic emotions that fuel the urgency to repeat the pathological use of the addictive-object. It is essential that the therapist make contact – without succumbing to terror – with the dissociated emotional contents involved in the addictive process. When reactivated within the therapeutic relationship, traumatic emotions do not remain confined to the patient's intrapsychic experience but permeate the relationship and the entire therapeutic field. In this context, enactment represents a crucial clinical juncture: recognizing it enables the therapist not only to orient themselves within the relational dynamics at play, but also to use it as a privileged instrument of psychic understanding and transformation.

Enactment

The extensive literature on enactment has progressively clarified its nature and core characteristics, showing that it is an eminently relational process that does not primarily involve the dynamic or repressed unconscious of analyst and patient, but rather the unrepressed and dissociated unconscious of both members of the dyad.

Despite the richness of theoretical contributions, enactment does not lend itself to a single, univocal definition: some authors conceptualize it as a particular form of procedural countertransference, while others emphasize its intersubjective and embodied dimensions. In my view, it is above all the work of Philip Bromberg that has convincingly clarified the specificity of enactment, freeing it from conceptual ambiguities and highlighting its not merely processual but profoundly relational and traumatic nature.

According to Bromberg (2011), enactment takes shape within what he describes as a dissociative cocoon, an interpersonal space in which therapist and patient are temporarily bound together through a dissociated mode of relating. He defines enactment as:

> a dyadic event in which therapist and patient are linked through a dissociated mode of relating, each in a 'not-me' state of his own that is affectively responsive to that of the other. This shared dissociative cocoon has its own imperative; it enmeshes and at least for a time traps the two partners within a 'not-me' communication field that is mediated by dissociation. In short, enactment is an intrapsychic phenomenon that is played out interpersonally, and it is through this interpersonal engagement that 'not-me' comes to be symbolically processed as 'me', a relational aspect of selfhood
>
> (pp. 151–52).

From this perspective, enactment can be understood as the outcome of a shared, unconscious (unrepressed) participation, in which the patient's unsymbolized traumatic memories are enacted and communicated to the analyst.

In my book *Enactment in the Therapeutic Relationship*, I have argued that, unlike transferential–countertransferential dynamics – which can be understood as the enactment of symbolic contents, mobilizing elements of the dynamic unconscious of both participants – enactment involves the acting out of the patient's dissociated traumatic experience, which is communicated implicitly and non-verbally to the analyst (Craparo, 2017). This communication occurs through the mechanism of projective identification and manifests in the therapist as intense bodily sensations, sudden emotional states, confusion, or temporary arrests of thought, mirroring the traumatic content evacuated by the patient into the therapeutic relationship.

Patient and therapist thus become involved in a shared dissociative condition, albeit in qualitatively different ways: in the patient, dissociation reflects a structural disaggregation of personality, whereas in the therapist it takes the form of a transient dissociative blackout, in which the body momentarily overrides reflective and symbolizing functions.

It should be emphasized that enactment is not in itself a pathological process, although it carries destabilizing potential. On the contrary, it may represent a valuable clinical opportunity insofar as it allows the therapist to come into direct contact with aspects of the patient's self that have not yet gained access to symbolic representation (Stern, 1997). However, for an experience to be recognized as enactment, it is essential that the therapist subsequently regains the capacity to reflect upon what is occurring within the therapeutic process.

In such moments, a calibrated and mentalized form of therapist self-disclosure (Craparo, 2024) may facilitate an initial transformative movement, gradually rendering thinkable what was initially only enacted.

Integrating enactment with Porges' Polyvagal Theory offers an additional level of understanding of this phenomenon. When viewed through the lens of autonomic nervous system functioning, enactment may be understood as a moment in which, during intense traumatic reactivation, both patient and therapist temporarily exit the domain of the ventral vagal system – responsible for social engagement, affect regulation, and mentalization. The therapeutic dyad thus enters an autonomic state oriented towards protection, dominated by sympathetic activation or dorsal vagal shutdown. In this condition, the body signals danger, reflective thinking diminishes, and the relationship becomes organized around survival responses.

Enactment may therefore be conceptualized as an *autonomic dissociative cocoon* (Figure 11.1), in which neurobiological responses to threat temporarily prevail over the capacity to mentalize.

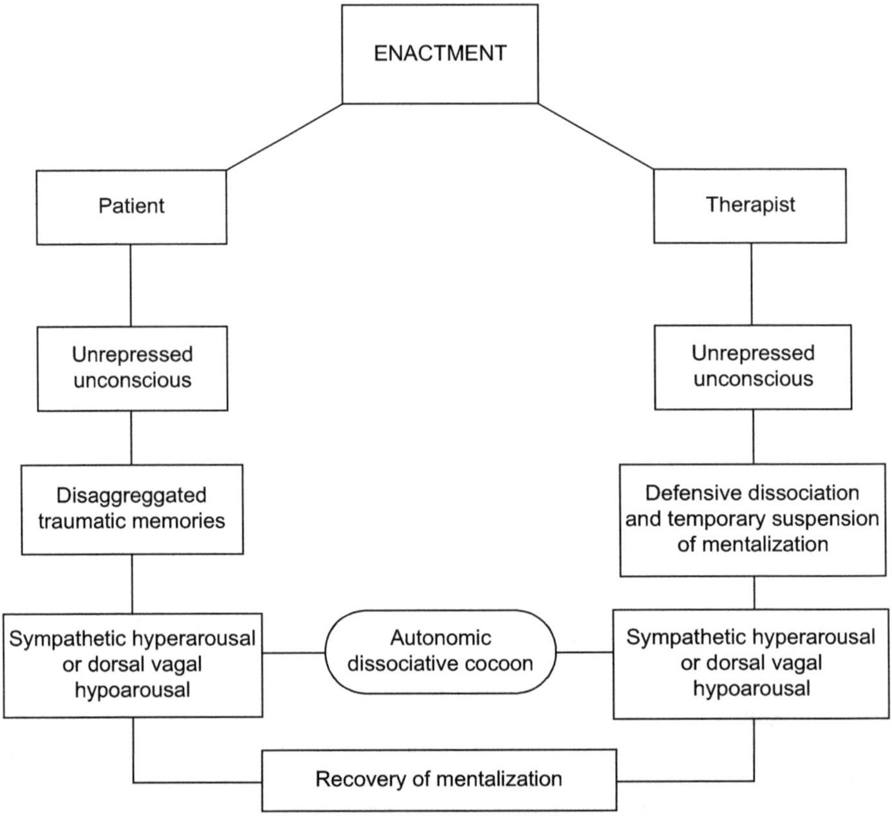

Figure 11.1 Enactment as an autonomic dissociative cocoon

It is crucial that the therapist facilitates a return to ventral vagal regulation, reactivating the conditions of safety necessary for what has been enacted to be symbolized, thought about, integrated into the patient's sense of self, and shared within a relational narrative.

The case of Arturo illustrates this dynamic in an emblematic way. Arturo (Craparo, 2017), an HIV-positive heroin user with a low-functioning borderline personality organization, entered therapy following panic attacks that emerged after the end of a significant romantic relationship. His developmental history is marked by severe early emotional deprivation and traumatic attachments, within a family context characterized by emotional absence, affective confusion, and early exposure to loss.

Throughout therapy, Arturo displayed marked anaffectivity, interrupted only when speaking about his former partner, at which point emotional activation became evident. During one session, he recounted a particularly bleak dream filled with images of degradation, destruction, and violence. The manner in which the dream was narrated elicited an intense bodily response in the therapist: a sense of malaise, a buzzing sensation in the head, and a progressive inability to think.

At that moment, Arturo's dissociated traumatic content was evacuated into the relationship and temporarily embodied by the therapist, who experienced a mind–body dissociation (a somatoform dissociation). In other words, the unrepressed unconscious of both patient and therapist communicated reciprocally, allowing the patient's traumatic memories to circulate within the therapeutic field and intertwine with the clinician's dissociative response.

Enactment thus took shape as a shared experience in which dissociation extended beyond the dyad to involve the entire embodied therapeutic setting (Lemma, 2014). From a polyvagal perspective, one might say that during the communication of traumatic memories, the therapeutic field temporarily exits a state of ventral vagal safety.

It is precisely the recognition of this temporary collusion, followed by the recovery of reflective functioning, that allows the therapist to transform enactment from a potential impasse into a clinical opportunity. By returning to Arturo, in an empathic and containing manner, the emotional meaning of the violent and primitive images populating the dream, the therapist contributed to the co-construction of an intersubjective space in which the traumatic experience could begin to be thought about – first and foremost by the therapist, who possessed an intact reality-testing capacity and mentalizing function – rather than merely enacted.

Enactment thus represents a delicate yet potentially fertile moment in therapeutic work with patients suffering from addiction; for this potential to be realized, however, the therapist must be able to recognize, sustain, and transform it.

Helping the Patient to Regulate Affects

In the opening chapters of this book, I have argued that, from a psychoanalytic perspective, what torments the addicted patient is an *internal Terrifying* – a force capable of evoking traumatic pain, that is, pain rooted in somatic states that precipitate the patient into a pervasive psychic malaise. It is from this state that the patient seeks escape by taking refuge in the compulsive use of one or more addictive-objects. In these patients, deficits in mentalization are closely correlated with affect dysregulation.

The therapeutic relationship, by working on the transformation of affective contents – contents that are somatically known but not thought, that is, not or only partially symbolically represented – embedded in traumatic memories, promotes the development of affect regulation. By affect regulation I refer to the identification, naming, recognition, and modulation of affective states. Empirical research has confirmed that the more developed a patient's capacity to mentalize affects, the lower the impact of craving.

Multilevel Intervention

Despite the central role of traumatic memories and the function of drugs as forms of self-medication, the treatment of addictive states requires multilevel interventions that take into account three main groups of variables:

1. Variables related to the characteristics of the addictive-object, including its chemical properties in the case of psychoactive substances, patterns and modalities of use (mono-use or poly-use), and the role of craving, sustained by hyperactivated memory and reward systems, which may re-emerge even after prolonged periods of abstinence.
2. Variables related to personality organization. In these patients, one does not encounter a specific 'addictive personality', but rather a frequent overlap with borderline and psychotic personality organizations. Impulsivity, identity diffusion, intense rage, experiences of emptiness and shame, and the re-enactment of traumatic relationships constitute core elements of the clinical work.
3. Variables related to treatment, which require:
   - stability of the setting as a temporal and symbolic anchor;
   - technical flexibility oriented primarily towards supportive interventions;
   - increased therapist activity (for example, through self-disclosure);
   - a high tolerance for hostility and the activation of primitive object relations;
   - discouragement of self-destructive behaviours;
   - careful monitoring of enactment and countertransference;
   - promotion of reflective functioning and mentalization;
   - development of affect regulation capacities;
   - facilitation of processes of integration of dissociated parts of the self.

From this perspective, psychotherapy for addiction may be understood as work aimed at restoring psychic continuity, experiential integration, and the capacity to desire, within a relational matrix that is sufficiently stable and empathic.

To situate addictions within the domain of dissociative trauma disorders explicitly entails orienting treatment towards work with traumatic memories. From this standpoint, I will outline several essential clinical nodes of an integrated treatment approach.

A first fundamental element concerns the recognition of the pain underlying addiction. Prior to any technical strategy, it is essential to be able to listen to and legitimize the suffering that the patient attempts to anaesthetize or keep at bay through compulsive behaviour. As described, addiction is not merely a symptom to be eliminated, but also a form of implicit communication – an embodied message that refers to a history of unprocessed pain. To intercept this suffering and to offer it a space of recognition and meaning-making constitutes the first step of any genuinely effective intervention.

A second key node involves the integration of a trauma- and dissociation-informed clinical perspective. The treatment of addiction cannot be separated from an awareness of the impact that early, dissociated, and non-mentalized traumatic experiences have on personality organization. This requires the adoption of clinical tools and a therapeutic stance capable of recognizing the fragmentation of the self, the activation of traumatic memories, dissociative phenomena, and the defensive strategies deployed by the patient in an attempt to survive internal states experienced as threatening or unbearable.

A further central axis concerns the construction of a sufficiently secure and reparative therapeutic alliance. In patients with histories of traumatic attachment (de Zulueta et al., 2025), basic trust is often profoundly compromised; as a result, the therapeutic relationship itself assumes an attachment function. The therapist is called upon to position themselves as an empathic, stable, and reliable presence, capable of offering a new affective experience that is non-judgemental and regulating. Within this relational frame, the patient may gradually begin to perceive themselves not exclusively through the lens of trauma, but also in terms of resources, resilience, and the possibility of change.

A fourth crucial point concerns the use of bottom-up interventions oriented towards the affective and somatic reworking of traumatic and addictive memories. The integration of techniques focused on bodily experience and on physiological and affective states enables non-verbal access to dissociated experiences, particularly where language and symbolic reflection are initially inaccessible. Through this kind of work, the patient can develop a greater awareness of internal states and self-regulatory capacities that progressively reduce the need to resort to the addictive-object as a protective strategy in the face of intense and threatening emotional activation. From this perspective, treatment fulfils a corrective function in relation to a distorted form of procedural learning.

Another important point involves the promotion of the capacity to mentalize the affective states implicated in addictive behaviours. More specifically, clinical work should support the transition from pre-mentalizing modes of functioning – in which affect is acted out, evacuated, or somatized – to modes in which emotional experience can be thought about, represented, and shared. It is precisely when the patient begins to name affects, rather than attempting to silence them through compulsive enactment, that an intersubjective space opens up – one that allows the emotional understanding of self and other and expands new possibilities for choice and transformation.

For this intersubjective space to emerge, however, it is necessary to work towards the integration of dissociated memories, so as to prevent unprocessed traumatic contents from persisting as unsymbolized fragments prone to invasive and disorganizing reactivation. The process of elaborating and integrating traumatic memories – through relational containment and narrative co-construction – makes it possible to place such experiences within a more coherent and tolerable autobiographical framework. This is a long and delicate process, requiring a solid therapeutic alliance, through which the patient can transform traumatic memory into recollection[1] – painful and disturbing, yet no longer traumatic. In this way, compulsive pressure is reduced and the maturation of a more integrated and self-aware subjectivity is facilitated.

I have outlined a number of trajectories that dynamically intertwine throughout the therapeutic process, modulating themselves according to the clinical moment, the patient's level of integration, and oscillations between states of regulation and dissociation. What unites these lines of work is their shared aim of accompanying the patient towards a fundamental goal: moving from the necessity to survive through dissociative and compulsive strategies to the possibility of living one's emotional and relational life in a full, creative, and safe (ventral-vagal) manner.

Note

1 With the term *memory* I refer to the implicit, sensory, and procedural reactivation of bodily experiences, whereas *recollection* refers to the explicit recall of events and mental states that have reached a level of elaboration such that they can be brought into the subject's awareness.

Chapter 12

An Integrated Approach to the Treatment of Addiction

In clinical work with patients suffering from addiction, the therapist is often permeated by the sense of being confronted with a fragility that, the deeper it is, the more it tends to express itself through marked resistance to the therapeutic process. Such resistance does not merely constitute an obstacle to clinical work; rather, it represents a structural feature of the patient's psychic functioning, one that continuously – and at times destabilizingly – questions the therapist's position.

In this regard, a scene from my early years as a therapist has remained particularly vivid in my mind. At the beginning of my clinical career, while working in an addiction service, I recall hearing the shouts of a psychiatrist colleague who, visibly overwhelmed, declared that she could no longer bear working with those patients and intended to request a transfer to a unit for psychotic patients. Even today, I can clearly picture that scene and the profound state of burnout in which she found herself – an expression of difficulty in containing and symbolizing the intense emotional demands coming from the patients, which had invaded the therapeutic relationship and the setting. What rendered the psychiatrist especially vulnerable to the patients' unconscious (unrepressed) communications was her failure to consider addiction in relation to underlying traumatic experiences, reducing addictions to dysfunctions of an essentially organic nature.

Over the years, I have learned to recognize not only the manipulative dimension often present in addicted patients – an integral part of their mental functioning – but also the crucial importance of the therapist maintaining a distance that is not emotional, but symbolic. Such distance is necessary in order not to be drawn into states of confusion that may lead, as in the psychiatrist's case, to withdrawal reactions or, in more severe situations, to far more problematic clinical and personal outcomes.

By distance I mean the therapist's capacity to preserve an adequate degree of separateness within an authentically intersubjective relationship. A separateness that allows the therapist to enter into a thinkable form of *collusion* with the patient's inner world, while avoiding the fusional *confusion* that abolishes difference and compromises the therapeutic function. In this sense,

DOI: 10.4324/9781003325314-13

maintaining relational asymmetry is fundamental: the therapist is called upon not to allow themselves to be captured by unconscious forces that might unwittingly entrap them within the patient's defences, thereby obstructing the possibility of transformative communication.

On closer inspection, it is precisely this separateness that makes it possible for the therapist to 'dream' the relationship with the patient, in Bion's sense of *rêverie*. To dream the patient and the relationship does not mean positioning oneself as the one who gives direction to the treatment (a lighthouse to be reached), but rather as a travelling companion who, holding a small lamp, helps to illuminate the path towards care and transformation.

To avoid misunderstandings, it is worth clarifying what I mean by collusion. Although the term is traditionally invoked in a predominantly negative sense – as an obstacle to the therapeutic relationship – collusion represents, in my view, a potential relational opportunity for the progress of clinical work, provided that the therapist is able to 'awaken' from that particular form of unconscious (especially unrepressed) reciprocal communication.

In this respect, Ronald Laing (1969) offers a particularly illuminating reflection on the meaning of the term collusion. He notes that the word shares the same linguistic root as delusion, illusion, and elusion. The root *lusion* derives from the past participle of the Latin verb *ludere*, whose meaning – both in classical and late Latin – includes playing, playing at something, engaging in sport, but also mocking and deceiving. Delusion thus implies not only the capacity to play, but also the possibility of self-deception, of illusion. Laing proposes using the term collusion while holding together both of these nuances: specifically, that of 'playing at' and that of 'deceiving'.

Collusion thus takes shape as a shared, intersubjective 'game', but also as a form of mutual deception. In work with addicted patients, collusion offers the therapist the opportunity to gain access to the patient's traumatic inner world; at the same time, however, it exposes the therapist to the risk of becoming entangled in it, slipping into a state of unconscious confusion that is not only emotional, but also concerns roles, with the consequent danger of violations of the therapeutic setting.

It is the analyst's responsibility to *awaken* from these deceptions – that is, to reflect upon the unconscious processes and mechanisms, both repressed and unrepressed, that structure the collusive experience. This entails recognizing that what is occurring in the here-and-now of the session represents a re-enactment – in the case of addicted patients – of traumatic memories and associated dissociative responses: namely, enactment.

It is within this horizon that the therapist is called upon to accompany the patient in the slow and patient co-construction of a transitional space: a shared and protected place in which what has long remained suffocated, feared, or unsayable can finally find welcome. Within this space, the most fragile and terrorized mental states gradually begin to take shape and find words, entering into a new and creative circuit of experience and meaning-making. Thus, the possibility opens up for a different narrative: a narrative of the self, of the other, and of the bond that connects them, but also of one's relationship with time – with a past that weighs heavily, with a present that slowly takes form, and with a future that becomes thinkable once again. The patient may then feel, for the first time, an active participant in a personal life project that is no longer merely endured, but progressively chosen and inhabited.

In this process, the therapist is required to give voice to their own humanity, so that the patient's humiliated humanity may be stirred and recognized. This appeal to the therapist's humanity cannot be separated from their capacity to engage fruitfully with their own vulnerability – a vulnerability that must neither be denied nor acted out, but rather integrated within technical attitudes capable of orienting and sustaining the therapeutic relationship. A relationship that may then be conceived as a dance, in which two subjectivities meet and, through their reciprocal movement, make possible the creation of something new and unprecedented within the patient's inner world.

An Integrated Trauma-Informed Treatment Model of Addictions

As Maté (2008) rightly suggests, believing that one can be effective through therapeutic work carried out in isolation with the patient is largely illusory. A multilevel approach is required – one that takes into account the specific characteristics of the addictive-object, considers the potential role of pharmacological interventions, and includes attention to the family context (given that the patient's trauma is often the legacy of transgenerational trauma).

With regard to psychological work with the patient, as I have argued throughout this book, it is not possible to dispense with work on traumatic memories (see Figure 12.1).

The therapeutic pathway in addictions is an integrated and dynamic process, articulated through interdependent and often overlapping phases, whose course is shaped by the level of personality organization, the presence of dissociation, and the function that addictive behaviour fulfils in the patient's somato-psychic life. The aim is not merely the elimination of the symptom, but the progressive transformation of the underlying mode of functioning that sustains it.

The work begins with a phase of in-depth clinical assessment, which goes beyond descriptive diagnosis and seeks to understand personality structure, traumatic history, modes of affect regulation, and the subjective meaning of the addictive-object or addictive behaviour. In parallel, the construction of the therapeutic alliance is initiated, as this represents the true foundation of treatment. In patients with addictions, relationships have often been the site of experiences of intrusion, abandonment, or violence; for this reason, trust cannot be taken for granted. It must be built over time through the consistency of the setting, the clarity of boundaries, and the therapist's capacity

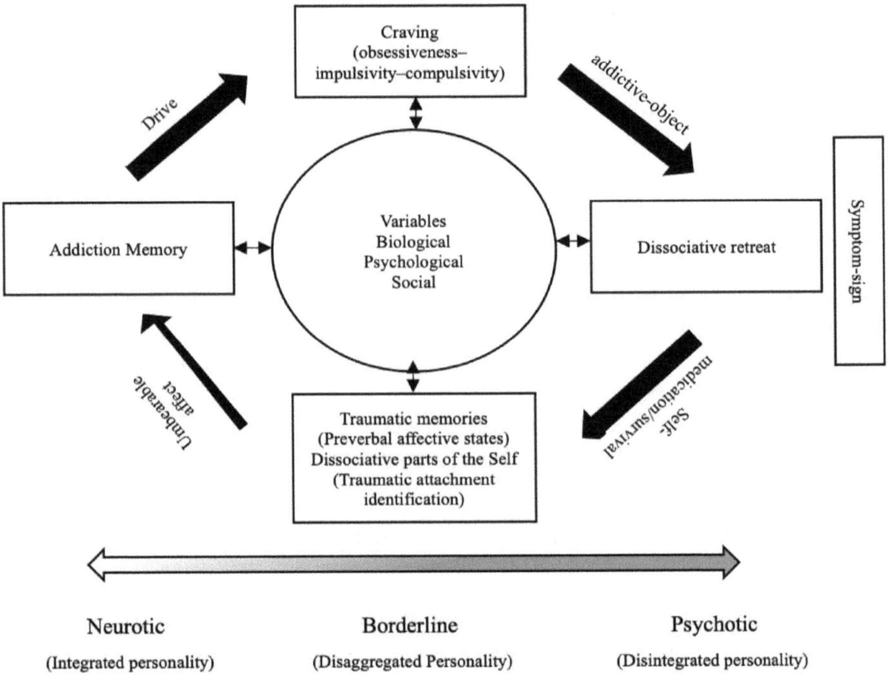

Figure 12.1 An integrated trauma-informed treatment model of addictions

to tolerate ambivalence, mistrust, and oscillations without colluding with addictive functioning or withdrawing emotionally.

Within this relational framework, it becomes possible to introduce psychoeducational work and reflective awareness of the addictive symptom. The patient is supported in understanding how continued substance use or compulsive behaviour interferes with the therapeutic process and with the possibility of coming into contact with internal states. This step does not serve a prescriptive or moralizing function. Rather, its aim is to foster an initial differentiation between the need for relief and the automatic behaviour that follows from it, making the psychological and relational costs of addiction thinkable. Where necessary, clinical work is integrated with medical or psychiatric interventions, particularly during phases of heightened instability.

Once minimal conditions of safety have been established, treatment can move towards stabilization and work with the body. Before any direct access to traumatic memories, it is essential that the patient develops a greater capacity to tolerate and recognize states of activation. Attention to bodily sensations associated with craving and compulsive use allows, over time, a reduction in the automatization of the act and brings the experience back into an intersubjective space. Sensations initially experienced as threatening or chaotic can thus be gradually named, shared, and placed within a meaningful framework.

At this stage of treatment, Focusing techniques encourage social engagement and co-regulation, supporting a sufficiently safe relational experience within which the patient can explore their inner world. This work involves an integrated engagement of the right and left hemispheres of the brain, proceeding in a bottom-up to top-down direction – that is, from implicit, bodily experience towards progressive explicitation and symbolization. Through this process, the patient is gradually supported in expanding an awareness of dissociated contents belonging to the unrepressed unconscious, often expressed in the form of bodily sensations, impulses, or affective states that are difficult to name.

Focusing thus facilitates a progressive process of familiarization with the body and with autonomic nervous system functioning, which in patients with trauma and addiction is frequently experienced as unpredictable or threatening. Drawing on Gendlin's original insights (1978/1981), Focusing is conceptualized as a contemplative practice primarily centred on immediate bodily experience rather than on the cognitive meaning of words. As Gendlin emphasized, the sense guiding the therapeutic process is initially non-conceptual; it emerges from the body as a global quality of experience that can be listened to and respected before it is understood.

In this direction, the contribution of Jan Winhall (2021) is particularly relevant. By integrating Focusing within the Felt Sense Polyvagal Model (FSPM), Winhall proposes a clinical approach sensitive to autonomic nervous system dynamics. She defines the felt sense as "a bodily knowing that can be subtle at first but opens up more and more as one gently attends to it" (Winhall, 2021, p. 2). The FSPM unfolds in phases and aims to stimulate a progressive experience of safety through changes in bodily felt experience. The clinical goal is not the suppression of activation states but the development of the capacity to recognize, tolerate, and modulate them more adaptively. In this way, the patient can gradually exit the vicious cycle of chronic alarm, which persists even in the absence of real danger, and develop greater flexibility in regulating internal responses to environmental demands.

Only when the patient has acquired sufficient stabilizing resources can the work orient towards a gradual access to traumatic memories and to the dissociated parts of the Self in which they are held. This transition takes place with respect for the window of tolerance, avoiding massive reactivations that would risk reinforcing recourse to dissociative retreat. The focus is not so much on a detailed reconstruction of traumatic events, but on the affective, bodily, and relational states that continue to be activated in the present.

At this stage, work on traumatic attachment becomes essential. Felicity de Zulueta (2025) developed the Traumatic Attachment Induction Procedure (TAIP) for the treatment of conditions related to traumatic attachment, including addictions. TAIP emerged from clinical observation of what occurs when, in the earliest stages of development, a child experiences fear, abuse, or neglect at the hands of the very figure upon whom survival entirely depends.

Under such conditions, the vital need to preserve the attachment bond is so absolute that the traumatic experience cannot be recognized or mentalized. In order to survive, the child is forced to 'forget', to split terror and pain off from conscious experience, while preserving an idealized image of the attachment figure. Although this solution is adaptive and life-preserving, it carries a profound cost: fragmentation of the Self and the formation of an unconscious traumatic attachment that continues to operate silently throughout life.

TAIP is positioned precisely at this nodal point of psychic functioning. Through a brief and highly focused procedure, it allows for the controlled evocation of the original traumatic attachment, rendering accessible the dissociated emotional and bodily responses that constitute its core. At the same time, TAIP works to deactivate the dissociative function of this attachment, fostering a more integrated encounter between parts of the Self that were forced to separate in order to ensure survival. The application of this procedure has shown promise in work with addictions, complicated grief, and other complex psychopathological conditions in which traumatic attachment continues to organize behaviour, relationships, and affect regulation. By offering direct, embodied access to these early nuclei, TAIP restores to the patient the possibility of transforming a bond originally founded on terror into an experience that can be recognized, processed, and integrated, opening the way towards a therapeutic process oriented towards continuity of the Self and the recovery of well-being (https://taip.uk).

Progressive contact with memories of traumatic attachment supports an integrative process sustained by the development of affective mentalization capacities. The patient begins to recognize, differentiate, and modulate emotional states, reducing the need to resort to the addictive-object in order to anaesthetize or contain them.

Conclusions

Enhancing mentalization capacity, developing skills for identifying and exploring traumatic emotions, working with current mental states, and fostering the possibility of inhabiting one's body constitute the fundamental stages of a therapeutic pathway oriented both towards the consolidation of change and relapse prevention. This involves accompanying the patient towards a deeper understanding of the emotional nature of addictive syndromes, helping them to view these not merely as dysfunctional behaviours, but as modes of regulating complex and non-mentalized affective states.

It thus becomes essential to support the patient in recognizing and naming these affective states, promoting ongoing reflection on the emotions that have traversed their past history, that are reactivated in the present through addictive compulsions, and that take shape in the *here and now* of the therapeutic relationship. Particular attention is given to implicit affective experiences organized around post-traumatic symptoms – such as shame, anger, humiliation, helplessness, and inefficacy – gradually supporting their mentalization and integration into the patient's conscious experience.

In parallel, clinical work requires that the therapist be able to tolerate and contain the patient's mental states within their own mind, maintaining constant attention to transferential, countertransferential, and enactment dynamics that permeate the therapeutic relationship. Within a sufficiently safe setting, the patient is thus accompanied in an integrative movement that allows, on the one hand, the processing of traumatic memories and, on the other, the reconstruction of greater continuity of experience and sense of Self.

Especially in the early phases of treatment – particularly in private practice settings rather than structured environments such as therapeutic communities – it is crucial that relapses are not read as failures, but as clinically meaningful signals of the reactivation of intense affective states or still-fragile dissociated parts. In this sense, the patient is helped to recognize such signals early and to draw upon alternative modes of affect regulation that have been built and consolidated throughout the course of treatment.

The ultimate aim of therapy is not the definitive elimination of the patient's vulnerabilities. Rather, it is to make possible a life no longer organized around addiction, but capable of including fragility without being dominated by it. From this perspective, therapeutic work enables the patient to recognize the 'monkey on one's back' as part of their personal history and past functioning – no longer an inevitable destiny, but something that can be known, contained, and ultimately overcome.

Chapter 13

Feeling Alive and Being Alive

I imagine the therapeutic relationship as a dance which, when it manages to find its own rhythm, becomes capable of fostering authentic change and generating something new and unprecedented, both for the patient and for the therapist. The metaphor of the dance is not incidental: it evokes a shared movement, an alternation of closeness and distance, and a continuous process of mutual regulation that can neither be fully planned nor left entirely to chance. Every dance, in order to unfold, requires minimal conditions that make it possible: a space, a time, and a symbolic frame that supports movement without rigidifying it.

In the same way, therapy requires fundamental preconditions in order to develop in a vital and effective manner. Among these, I consider central – as already mentioned – the co-construction of *spacing* (Nancy, 1996), understood as a symbolic, psychic, and intersubjective space that is not guaranteed solely by role differentiation, but above all by the therapeutic function that the clinician is called upon to assume, embody, and maintain over time (Craparo, 2025). Spacing does not simply coincide with the setting in its formal sense but represents a deeper dimension: a mental field that allows for the suspension of enactment, the transformation of experience, and the emergence of thought.

It is from this function that the asymmetry of the therapeutic relationship takes shape. An asymmetry that should not be understood as emotional distance, impersonal neutrality, or a position of epistemic superiority, but rather as a specific mode of emotional participation and clinical responsibility. The therapist is not 'above' the patient, nor positioned outside the relationship; on the contrary, they are fully involved, yet in a position that enables them to sustain the field and guarantee its continuity. Asymmetry thus concerns function, not the value of subjectivity: both are present as persons, but with different tasks.

It is the therapist's responsibility to offer a place capable of welcoming the patient's demand: a sufficiently safe context within which a process can be undertaken that involves exposure, risk, commitment, and effort for both parties. Entering therapy means, for the patient, exposing themselves to a

DOI: 10.4324/9781003325314-14

relationship that inevitably reactivates affective memories, expectations, fears, and deep desires; it also means confronting what has been avoided, anaesthetized, or dissociated. For this to occur without producing further traumatization, it is necessary that the setting be experienced as reliable and that the therapist can function as the guarantor of the field's stability.

In this sense, the personality of the therapist – just like that of the patient – becomes an integral part of the therapeutic process. This entails moving beyond the abstract and impracticable notion of anonymity that long dominated certain conceptions of analytic technique. Far from being an external, distant, and anonymous observer, the therapist participates in the relationship with the entirety of their being: feelings, beliefs, thoughts, motivations, memories, and life experiences inevitably enter the therapeutic field. Not as elements to be displayed or imposed, but as silent and active components of an intersubjective process that thereby acquires genuine transformative power.

The therapeutic field is never a neutral surface: it is a densely inhabited place in which histories, fantasies, expectations, and lived experiences belonging to both members of the dyad intertwine. Recognizing this dimension does not mean relinquishing the therapeutic function; on the contrary, it strengthens it, as it allows the therapist to adopt a reflective position towards what occurs in the relationship, rather than unconsciously enacting their own emotional resonances.

This relational field is nourished by the therapist's authenticity and their capacity for sensitive and responsive listening. A form of listening that is not limited to a cognitive understanding of the patient's discourse but that addresses their otherness, attuning to their inner world and to what has not yet found a representable form. It involves a willingness to be affected, to resonate emotionally with the patient's unconscious (unrepressed) contents, without losing the transformative function that characterizes therapeutic work. It is precisely within this unstable balance between participation and function that the therapeutic relationship can remain alive and generative.

The reference is inevitably to Ogden's notion of "dreaming the patient's undreamt or interrupted dreams", so that the patient may gradually reclaim them. From this perspective, the therapist temporarily lends their capacity to dream, to think and to mentalize, offering the patient a space in which traumatic experiences that have remained unformulated can begin to be symbolized. Dreaming, in this sense, is not a strictly oneiric activity, but a psychic function that enables the transformation of raw experience into thinkable material: here the reference is to what Bion (1962) wrote about the analyst's capacity for *rêverie.*

The ultimate aim is not merely symptom reduction or the elimination of distress, but to help the patient *feel real,* to experience an authentic, living, human Self. Many patients come to therapy with the sense of not fully existing, of living in a condition of psychic survival, in which contact with desire has been replaced by defensive strategies of control, anaesthesia or enactment.

Therapeutic work thus seeks to restore to the subject the possibility of inhabiting their own experience, recognizing it as their own, and thereby learning *to play with reality.*

Just as in early development play within the intersubjective caregiver–child relationship plays a decisive role in the process of humanization and in the consolidation of a real Self, so too in therapy it is necessary for the clinician to be willing to play and to dream with the patient. I understand play as an essential function that allows reality to be explored without being overwhelmed by it, to experiment with new configurations of experience and to tolerate uncertainty. In this sense, dreaming is playing and playing is dreaming: both are processes that allow traumatic experience to be revisited and new narrative possibilities to be generated.

Within therapeutic play, the patient can experience a relationship in which the other is neither intrusive nor withdrawn, but present in a sufficiently safe way. This experience, repeated over time, enables the construction of a sense of Self-continuity and the emergence of a basic trust in relationship. It is here that therapy takes shape as a transformative environment, capable of fostering not only understanding, but above all corrective emotional experience.

As one patient who had benefited from our work once told me: "Psychotherapy is a mental environment in which my desire can proliferate. An environment that fosters an inner dialogue capable of nourishing my desire to live." This statement captures with great precision the profound aim of clinical work: not so much to 'fix' what is not working, but to create the conditions for desire to begin to circulate. Therapy thus becomes a Third space in which the subject can withdraw from compulsive repetition and open themselves to unprecedented forms of experience.

Along this path, the patient may develop an aesthetic feeling never previously experienced: a new sensitivity that makes beauty perceptible even where there was previously only pain, emptiness, or emotional anaesthesia. I understand the aesthetic feeling not in an ornamental sense, but as a mode of relating to experience that involves involvement, resonance, and the capacity to be affected. It is a form of pleasure that arises from encountering meaning, from recognizing one's own experience as endowed with value.

If we reflect on it, aesthetics has to do with human sensibility, as suggested by the Greek term *aisthesis*, which refers to sensation and feeling. The aesthetic feeling is one of pleasure and admiration, an integral part of the poetic dimension of existence (Morin, 2016). Beauty, from this perspective, resides not so much in the object as in the quality of pleasure it evokes, in its capacity to set desire in motion. Beauty lives in the gaze of the beholder, in the ability to allow oneself to be involved in experience without reducing it to function or performance.

Healing thus takes shape as the possibility of accessing an aesthetic feeling that allows the patient to tolerate pain and attribute meaning to it – transforming trauma into a psychic and relational plot – while at the same time opening to the time of enjoyment, pleasure and desire. Healing does not mean eliminating suffering, but being able to integrate it into a broader narrative in which life becomes inhabitable once again.

Perhaps it is here that the metaphor of the dance finds its fulfilment: movement is no longer imposed by traumatic repetition, but arises from a rediscovered capacity to feel, choose, and desire; the patient can finally participate in their own experience, no longer as a distant spectator or an anaesthetized body, but as a living presence in the world.

The Limit of Care as a Condition of Transformative Experience

Affirming the possibility of change, of a reopening of desire and of renewed vitality does not mean ignoring the intrinsic limits of therapeutic work with patients who present histories of complex trauma and profound dissociative functioning. On the contrary, recognizing the limits of care constitutes an indispensable condition for psychotherapy not to turn into an implicit promise of salvation – one that is all the more fragile the more silent it remains. Not all patients are able to make the transition from survival to life, from dissociative withdrawal to a more integrated subjective experience; nor can the impossibility of this transition always be traced back to technical error or lack of commitment. If, for instance, we imagine that we can turn an adult psychotic patient into a neurotic one, we introduce a bias that leads us to attribute to the patient competencies and possibilities for improvement that are not achievable.

I believe that the therapist's task does not coincide with guaranteeing a fully transformative outcome, but with keeping open a psychic space in which the patient's experience can be welcomed and thought about, even when change remains partial or uncertain. There are trajectories in which the greatest attainable result consists in a reduction of destructiveness, a greater awareness of internal states, or simply the possibility of not being alone with one's pain. These achievements, seemingly minimal, may at times represent decisive gains in relation to functioning dominated by dissociation and enactment.

Thinking about the limits of care allows therapeutic work with addiction to be freed from any redemptive rhetoric and restores its profoundly human dimension: a practice exposed to uncertainty, risk and the unpredictability of encounter. It is precisely by accepting this uncertainty that the therapeutic relationship can maintain its authenticity and continue to offer – even in the most complex cases – not the promise of absolute healing, but the possibility of a meaningful experience. And it is from this fragile, partial possibility that a new way of feeling oneself and the world may sometimes emerge for the patient, opening space for unprecedented forms of participation in life.

Chapter 14

Concluding Remarks

Throughout this volume I have proposed understanding addictions not as disorders of the object, nor as simple behavioural deviations, but as complex configurations of psychic and somatic functioning, rooted in dissociative traumatic experiences and early failures of affect regulation. From this perspective, addictive behaviour loses its enigmatic or morally connoted character and reveals itself instead as an attempt at survival: an extreme, dysfunctional, yet necessary solution adopted by an organism that has found no other way to cope with overwhelming internal states.

Addiction, thus understood, is not the problem in itself, but the signal of a deeper problem. It is the visible expression of a malaise that has found in the body and in enactment its only possibility of manifestation. What the clinician encounters is not simply a subject who 'cannot stop', but a person whose developmental history is marked by relational trauma, experiences of misattunement, and non-integrated implicit memories that continue to act in the present as if danger were still current.

This reading allows us to move beyond one of the most sterile dichotomies that have traversed the field of addictions: that of biological vs psychodynamic models. The neurobiological processes involved in addiction – from dysfunctions of reward circuits to allostasis, from stress-system dysregulation to impairment of executive functions – are not alternatives to psychological and relational processes, but their embodied correlates. The body, in other words, is the theatre in which the subject's relational history has been inscribed in the form of somato-psychic memory.

In this sense, the concept of dissociative withdrawal acquires central clinical and heuristic value. The use of the addictive-object, as well as the enactment of compulsive behaviours, can be understood as a somato-psychic refuge: an internal dissociative space that allows escape from pain that cannot be thought or shared. Dissociative withdrawal is not merely an escape from reality but an escape into the reality of the body, where language has failed and relationship has been experienced as dangerous.

From this perspective, craving also loses its aura of mystery. It is not simply an uncontrollable impulse, but the expression of a primary regulatory need. It

DOI: 10.4324/9781003325314-15

is the voice of the body signalling a state of internal threat and urgently requesting an intervention capable of restoring a minimum threshold of tolerability. The fact that such intervention takes the form of a substance or harmful behaviour does not erase its original function: attempting to soothe a nervous system trapped in defence.

I believe that considering addictions as trauma-related disorders – and more precisely as expressions of dissociative trauma – has important clinical implications. First, it shifts the focus of intervention from mere cessation of behaviour to understanding the processes that sustain it. Asking a patient to stop using a substance without offering alternative forms of regulation often amounts to asking them to give up the only strategy they know to survive. It is therefore unsurprising that relapse is frequent when the symptom disappears without the underlying pain having found containment.

Truly effective treatment instead requires progressive work on multiple levels: safety, affect regulation, the therapeutic relationship, and the capacity to recognize and mentalize bodily and emotional states that were previously dissociated. The integrated model informed by dissociative trauma and affect regulation proposed in this book should not be understood as a rigid sequence of phases, but as a flexible framework that takes into account the patient's specific personality organization, the severity of dissociation, and the degree of impairment of reality testing.

In particular, the distinction between neurotic, borderline, and psychotic organizations allows the clinical intervention to be modulated, avoiding standardized approaches that risk being ineffective or iatrogenic.

A crucial aspect concerns the role of the therapist. Working with addictions means exposing oneself to intense dynamics, powerful enactments, and continuous oscillations between approach and withdrawal. It requires a clinical presence that is both secure and human, capable of tolerating impotence, frustration, and failure without resorting to defensive solutions such as control, judgement, or disengagement. The therapeutic relationship thus becomes a space of human experience in which the patient can encounter, sometimes for the first time, a sufficiently stable form of affective attunement.

Change is a slow process, marked by advances and relapses, partial integrations and new equilibria. Yet it is precisely within this gradualness that space opens for a life increasingly less dominated by urgency and more inhabitable by desire.

Ultimately, thinking about addictions in relation to the subject's traumatic history means restoring a possibility: that of understanding the meaning of one's suffering and of gradually constructing alternative ways of being with oneself and with others. It is in this direction that the clinic of addictions can rediscover its most authentically human dimension: that of accompanying a person in the difficult work of coming back to feeling alive.

The Dissociative Trauma and Affect Dysregulation Related Addiction Model

Since I conceptualize addictions as trauma-related disorders of a dissociative nature, I would like to clarify more explicitly how the *Dissociative Trauma and Affect Dysregulation Related Addiction Model* differs from other interpretative frameworks that have made significant contributions to understanding addiction. This comparison is not intended to establish theoretical hierarchies, but to highlight what this model allows us to understand more fully, or differently.

In relation to the self-medication hypothesis, the model moves beyond a predominantly functional reading of addictive behaviour. While acknowledging the role of psychic pain as an antecedent to use, the model proposes understanding craving not merely as the search for relief, but as the expression of a dissociative state organized around non-integrated implicit traumatic memories. From this perspective, addiction is not simply a strategy of self-medication, but a true somato-psychic reenactment of early traumatic experiences, inscribed in the body and reactivated in the present. This allows for a deeper understanding of loss of control, Self-fragmentation, and the alien and coercive quality of the impulse to use.

The model is situated within a developmental–relational framework. Traumatic relationships are not considered solely as experiences internalized at a representational level, but as events that directly affect autonomic nervous system regulation and the structuring of bodily memory. Addiction thus becomes a privileged modality through which these states find expression and regulation, outside the field of symbolization.

The model proposes an integrated reading that brings relational neurobiology, psychoanalysis, attachment theory and body-centred techniques into dialogue. It presents itself as an integrative framework that shifts the clinical focus from the object to the body, from behaviour to dissociation, from will to regulation. From this perspective, addiction is related to a body that continues to ask for safety, recognition, and presence.

If listened to without prejudice, addiction speaks not only of destruction, but of the extreme attempt of a body–mind to remain alive when all other paths have failed. It is from this understanding that therapeutic work with addicted patients can find its deepest meaning.

References

Albasi, C. (2006). *Attaccamenti traumatici: I modelli operativi interni dissociati.* Milano: Utet.

American Psychiatric Association. (2013). *Diagnostic and statistical manual of mental disorders* (5th ed.). American Psychiatric Publishing.

American Psychiatric Association. (2022). *Diagnostic and statistical manual of mental disorders* (5th ed., text rev.). American Psychiatric Publishing.

Beebe, B., & Lachmann, F. M. (2002). *Infant research and adult treatment: Co-constructing interactions.* London: The Analytic Press/Taylor & Francis Group.

Bion, W. R. (1962). *Learning from experience.* London: Karnac Books.

Boening, J. A. (2001). Neurobiology of an addiction memory. *Journal of Neural Transmission*, 108 (6), 755–765.

Bollas, C. (1987). *The shadow of the object: Psychoanalysis of the unthought known.* London: Free Association Books.

Bollas, C. (2019). *Forces of destiny. Psychoanalysis and human idiom.* London & New York: Routledge.

Bowlby, J. (1979). *The making and breaking of affectional bonds.* London: Tavistock Publications.

Bowlby, J. (1980). *Attachment and loss. vol. 3: Loss, sadness and depression.* New York: Basic Books.

Bowlby, J. (1988). *A secure base: Parent-child attachment and healthy human development.* New York: Basic Books.

Breslau, N. & Schultz, L. (2013). Neuroticism and post-traumatic stress disorder: a prospective investigation. *Psychological Medicine*, 43 (8), 1697–1702.

Bromberg, P. M. (1998). *Standing in the spaces: Essays on clinical process, trauma and dissociation.* Hillsdale, NJ: The Analytic Press.

Bromberg, P. M. (2001). Treating patients with symptoms – and symptoms with patience: Reflections on shame, dissociation, and eating disorders. *Psychoanalytic Dialogues*, 11 (6), 891–912.

Bromberg, P. M. (2006). *Awakening the dreamer: Clinical journeys.* London & New York: Routledge.

Bromberg, P. M. (2011). *The shadow of the tsunami and the growth of the relational mind.* London & New York: Routledge.

Bucci, W. (1997). *Psychoanalysis and cognitive science: A multiple code theory.* Guilford Press.

Burroughs, W. S. (1977). *Junky.* New York: Penguin Books.

Caretti, V. & Craparo, G. (2005). La correlazione tra alessitimia e dissociazione in un gruppo di tossicodipendenti. In V. Caretti & D. La Barbera (Eds.), *Alessitimia. Valutazione e trattamento.* Roma: Astrolabio.

Caretti, V. & Craparo, G. (Eds.). (2008). *Trauma e psicopatologia: Un approccio evolutivo-relazionale.* Roma: Astrolabio.

Caretti, V., Craparo, G., & Schimmenti, A. (2010). Fattori evolutivo-relazionali dell'addiction. Uno studio sulla dipendenza da eroina. In V. Caretti & D. La Barbera (Eds.), *Addiction. Aspetti biologici e di ricerca* (pp. 99–134). Milano: Raffaello Cortina.

Caretti, V., Craparo, G., Ragonese, N., & Schimmenti, A. (2005). Disregolazione affettiva, trauma e dissociazione in un gruppo non clinico di adolescenti: Una prospettiva evolutiva. *Infanzia e Adolescenza,* 3, 22–30.

Caretti, V., Craparo, G., & Schimmenti, A. (2006). Fattori di rischio della dipendenza patologica in adolescenza. *Infanzia e Adolescenza,* 3, 160–169.

Caretti, V., Craparo, G., Giannini, M., Gori, A., Iraci Sareri, G., Lucchini, A., Rusignuolo, I., & Schimmenti, A. (2016). *Addictive behavior questionnaire (ABQ): Manual and questionnaire.* Firenze: Hogrefe.

Caretti, V., Gori, A., Craparo, G., Giannini, M., Iraci-Sareri, G., & Schimmenti, A. (2018). A new measure for assessing substance-related and addictive disorders: The Addictive Behavior Questionnaire (ABQ). *Journal of Clinical Medicine,* 7 (8), 194. doi:10.3390/jcm7080194.

Chefetz, R. A. (2015). *Intensive psychotherapy for persistent dissociative processes: The fear of feeling real.* New York: W. W. Norton & Company.

Correale A. (2010), La difficile differenziazione dalla identificazione traumatica. La forza gravitazionale del trauma. *Comprendere,* 20, 52–65.

Craparo, G. (2008). La dipendenza sessuale: le emozioni traumatiche e la vulnerabilità al dolore. In V. Caretti, G. Craparo, & A. Schimmenti (Eds.), *Memorie traumatiche e mentalizzazione* (pp. 157–168). Roma: Astrolabio.

Craparo, G. (2013). *Il disturbo post-traumatico da stress.* Roma: Carocci.

Craparo, G. (2017). *L'enactment nella relazione terapeutica. Caratteristiche e funzioni.* Milano: Raffaello Cortina.

Craparo, G. (2018). *Inconscio non rimosso.* Milano: FrancoAngeli.

Craparo, G. (2024). *Menti che si svelano. Caratteristiche e funzioni.* Milano: FrancoAngeli.

Craparo, G. (2026). *Teoria e clinica del trauma dissociativo.* Firenze: Giunti.

Craparo, G., & Mucci, C. (Eds.). (2016). *Unrepressed unconscious, implicit memory, and clinical work.* London: Karnac.

Craparo, G., & Mucci, C. (Eds.). (2026). *Embodied psychoanalysis. Body, mind and relationship.* London & New York: Routledge.

De Masi, F. (2018). *Svelare l'enigma della psicosi: Fondamenti per una terapia analitica.* Milano: Mimesis.

De Zulueta, F., Notice, M., Unadkat, J., & de Escoriaza, L. (2025). *Healing the fractured mind: A revolutionary method for treating addiction and other disorders.* London: Karnac.

Di Ciaccia, A., & Recalcati, M. (2000). *Jacques Lacan.* Milano: Bruno Mondadori.

Dube, S. R., Anda, R. F., Felitti, V. J., Edwards, V. J., & Croft, J. B. (2002). Adverse childhood experiences and personal alcohol abuse as an adult. *Addictive Behaviors,* 27 (5), 713–725.

Duncan, L. E., Cooper, B. N., & Shen H. (2018). Robust findings from 25 years of PTSD genetics research. *Current Psychiatry Reports*, 20, article 115.

Edelman, G. (1989). *The remembered present: A biological theory of consciousness*. New York: Basic Books.

Fairbairn, W. R. D. (1952). *Psychoanalytic studies of the personality*. London: Routledge & Kegan Paul.

Fairbairn, W. R. D. (1963). Synopsis of an object-relations theory of the personality. *The International Journal of Psychoanalysis*, 44 (2), 224–225.

Farina, B., Liotti, M., Imperatori, C. (2019). The role of attachment trauma and disintegrative pathogenic processes in the traumatic-dissociative dimension. *Frontiers in Psychology*, 26, 10, 933.

Felitti, V. J., Anda, R. F., Nordenberg, D., Williamson, D. F., Spitz, A. M., Edwards, V., … Marks, J. S. (1998). Relationship of childhood abuse and household dysfunction to many of the leading causes of death in adults: The Adverse Childhood Experiences (ACE) Study. *American Journal of Preventive Medicine*, 14 (4), 245–258.

Ferenczi, S. (1949). Confusion of the tongues between the adults and the child – (The language of tenderness and of passion) 1932. *International Journal of Psychoanalysis*, 30, 225–230.

Fonagy, P., & Target, M. (1997). Attachment and reflective function: Their role in self-organization. *Development and Psychopathology*, 9 (4), 679–700.

Fonagy, P., Gergely, G., Jurist, E. L., & Target M. (2002). *Affect regulation, mentalization, and the development of the self*. New York, NY: Other Press.

Freud, S. (1900/1953). *The interpretation of dreams* (Standard Edition, Vol. 5). London: Hogarth Press.

Freud, S. (1919) The 'Uncanny'. In *The standard edition of the complete psychological works of Sigmund Freud*, vol XVII (pp. 217–256). London: Vintage.

Freud, S. (1920/1961). *Beyond the pleasure principle*. New York & London: W. W. Norton.

Freud, S. & Breuer, J. (1955). *The standard edition of the complete psychological works of Sigmund Freud, Volume II (1893–1895): Studies on hysteria*. London: Hogarth Press.

Gallese, V. (2014). Quali neuroscienze e quale psicoanalisi?: Intersoggettività e Sé corporeo: Appunti per un dialogo. *Rivista di Psicoanalisi* 60, 687–703.

Green, A. (1993). *The dead mother. Psyche*, 47(3), 205–240.

Janet, P. (1889). *Psychological automatism, vol. I & II*. London & New York: Routledge, 2021.

Janet, P. (1907). *The major symptoms of hysteria*. New York: Macmillan.

Janet, P. (1909). *Les névroses*. Ernest Flammarion.

Jurist, E. L. (2005). Mentalized affectivity. *Psychoanalytic Psychology*, 22 (3), 426–444.

Hao, F., Li, P., Liang, Z., & Geng, J. (2024). The association between childhood adverse experiences and internet addiction: A meta-analysis. *Acta Psychologica*, 246, 104270.

Hari, J. (2015). *Chasing the scream: The opposite of addiction is connection*. New York: Bloomsbury.

Howell, E. F. (2020). *Trauma and dissociation informed psychotherapy: Relational healing and the therapeutic connection*. New York: Norton.

Hughes, K., Bellis, M. A., Sethi, D., Andrew, R., Yon, Y., Wood, S., … Zakhozha, V. (2019). Adverse childhood experiences, childhood relationships and associated substance use and mental health in young Europeans. *European Journal of Public Health*, 29 (4), 741–747.

Kaës, R. (2012). *Le malêtre.* Paris: Dunod.

Kernberg, O. F. (1975). *Borderline conditions and pathological narcissism.* New York: Jason Aronson.

Kernberg, O. F. (1984). *Severe personality disorders: Psychotherapeutic strategies.* New Haven: Yale University.

Khantzian, E. J. (1985). The self-medication hypothesis of addictive disorders. *American Journal of Psychiatry,* 142 (11), 1259–1264.

Khantzian, E. J. (1997). The self-medication hypothesis of substance use disorders: A reconsideration and recent applications. *Harvard Review of Psychiatry,* 4 (5), 231–244.

Kohut, H. (1971). *The analysis of the self.* New York: International Universities Press.

Koob, G. F., & Bloom, F. E. (1988). Cellular and molecular mechanisms of drug dependence. *Science,* 242 (4879), 715–723.

Koob, G. F. & Volkow, N. D. (2016). Neurobiology of addiction: a neurocircuitry analysis. *Lancet Psychiatry,* 3 (8), 760–773.

Kotera, Y., & Rhodes, C. (2019). Pathways to sex addiction: Relationships with adverse childhood experience, attachment, narcissism, self-compassion and motivation in a gender-balanced sample. *Sexual Addiction and Compulsivity,* 26 (1–2), 54–76.

Lacan, J. (2020). *The seminar, Book IV: The object relation (1956/1957).* Cambridge and Medford MA: Polity Press.

Lacan, J. (2021). *Desire and its interpretation: The seminar of Jacques Lacan, Book VI (1958–1959).* Cambridge & Medford MA: Polity Press.

Laing, R. D. (1969). *Self and other.* London & New York: Routledge.

Lanius, U. F., Paulsen, S. L. & Corrigan, F. M. (Eds.) (2014). *Neurobiology and treatment of traumatic dissociation: Toward an embodied self.* New York: Springer Publishing Company.

Laplanche, J & Pontalis J-C. (2018). *The Language of psychoanalysis.* London & New York: Routledge.

Lemma, A. (2014). The body of the analyst and the analytic setting: reflections on the embodied setting and the symbiotic transference. *International Journal of Psychoanalysis,* 95 (2), 225–244.

Lewis, M. (2015). *The biology of desire: Why addiction is not a disease.* New York: PublicAffairs.

Leza, L., Siria, S., López-Goñi, J. J., & Fernández-Montalvo, J. (2021). Adverse childhood experiences (ACEs) and substance use disorder (SUD): A scoping review. *Drug and Alcohol Dependence,* 221, 108563.

Lighstone, J. (2004). Dissociation and compulsive eating. *Journal of Trauma and Dissociation,* 5 (4), 17–32.

Lingiardi, V. (2025). *Farsi male.* Torino: Einaudi.

Main, M. (1995). Recent studies in attachment: Overview, with selected implications for clinical work. In S. Goldberg, R. Muir & J. Kerr (Eds.), *Attachment theory: Social, developmental, and clinical perspectives* (pp. 407–474). New York: Analytic Press, Inc.

Maté, G. (2008). *In the realm of hungry ghosts: Close encounters with addiction.* North Atlantic Books.

Meares, R. (2012). *A dissociation model of borderline personality disorder.* W. W. Norton.

Milton, A. L., & Everitt, B. J. (2012). The persistence of maladaptive memory: Addiction, drug memories and anti-relapse treatments. *Neuroscience and Biobehavioral Reviews,* 36 (4), 1119–1139.

Modell, A. H. (1999). The dead mother syndrome and the reconstruction of trauma. In G. Kohon (Ed.). *The dead mother. The work of André Green* (pp. 76–87). London & New York: Routledge.

Morin, E. (2016). *Sur l'esthétique.* Paris: Èdition Robert Laffont.

Morison, M. & Benight, C. C. (2022). Trauma coping self-efficacy mediates associations between adult attachment and posttraumatic stress symptoms. *Frontiers in Psychology*, 7, 13, 799608.

Mucci, C. (2018). *Borderline bodies. Affect regulation therapy.* New York: W.W. Norton & Company.

Nancy, J. L. (1996). *Être singulier pluriel.* Lorainne: Galilée.

Nijenhuis, E. R. S. (2014). Ten reasons for conceiving and classifying posttraumatic stress disorder as a dissociative disorder. *Psichiatrica e Psicoterapia*, 33, 74–106.

Ogle, C. M., Rubin, D. C., & Siegler, I. C. (2013). The impact of the developmental timing of trauma exposure on PTSD symptoms and psychosocial functioning among older adults. *Developmental Psychology*, 49 (11), 2191–2200.

Pievani, T. (2017). *La teoria dell'evoluzione.* Bologna: il Mulino.

Pineles, S. L, Mostoufi, S. M., Ready, C. B., Street, A. E., Griffin, M. G., & Resick P. A. (2011). Trauma reactivity, avoidant coping, and PTSD symptoms: a moderating relationship? *Journal of Abnormal Psychology*, 120 (1), 240–246.

Porges, S. W. (2001). The polyvagal theory: Phylogenetic substrates of a social nervous system. *International Journal of Psychophysiology*, 42 (2), 123–146.

Porges, S. W. (2011). *The polyvagal theory: Neurophysiological foundations of emotions, attachment, communication, and self-regulation.* New York: W. W. Norton & Company.

Porges, S. W. (2022). Addiction: A polyvagal perspective. *International Body Psychotherapy Journal*, 21 (1), 13–16.

Putnam, F. (1997). *Dissociation in children and adolescents. A developmental perspective.* New York: Guilford Press.

Ramo-Fernández, L., Schneider, A., Wilker, S., & Kolassa, I. T. (2015). Epigenetic alterations associated with war trauma and childhood maltreatment. *Behavioral Sciences and Law*, 33 (5), 701–721.

Ross, T. A. (1941). *War neuroses.* Baltimore, MD: Williams & Wilkins.

Russell, M. & Barral, C. (2019). The holistic project of Pierre Janet. Part one: Disintegration or désagrégation. In G. Craparo, F. Ortu, & O. van der Hart (Eds.), *Rediscovering Pierre Janet. Trauma, dissociation, and a new context for psychoanalysis.* London & New York: Routledge.

Schemitsch, C. & Nauth A. (2019). Psychological factors and recovery from trauma. *Injury*, 51 (2), S64–S66.

Schore, A. N. (1994). *Affect regulation and the origin of the self: The neurobiology of emotional development.* Mahwah, NJ: Lawrence Erlbaum Associates, Inc.

Schore, A. N. (2001). The effects of early relational trauma on right brain development, affect regulation, and infant mental health. *Infant Mental Health Journal*, 22 (1–2), 201–269.

Schore, A. N. (2012). *The science of the art of psychotherapy.* W. W. Norton & Company.

Schore, A. N. (2015). *Affect regulation and the origin of the self: The neurobiology of emotional development.* London & New York: Routledge.

Sharma, A., & Sacco, P. (2015). Adverse childhood experiences and gambling: Results from a national survey. *Journal of Social Work Practice in the Addictions*, 15 (1), 25–43.

Shors, T. (2021). *Everyday trauma: Remapping the brain's response to stress, anxiety, and painful memories for a better life*. New York: Penguin Press.

Siegel, D. (1999). *The developing mind*. New York & London: The Guilford Press.

Siegel, D. J. (2010). *The mindful therapist: A clinician's guide to mindsight and neural integration*. New York: W. W. Norton & Company.

Steiner, J. (1993). *Psychic retreats: Pathological organizations in psychotic, neurotic and borderline patients*. London & New York: Routledge.

Stern, D. (1985). *The interpersonal world of the infant: A view from psychoanalysis and developmental psychology*. New York: Basic Books.

Stern, D. B. (1997). *Unformulated experience: From dissociation to imagination in psychoanalysis*. Hillsdale, NJ: The Analytic Press.

Taylor, G. J., Bagby, R. M., & Parker, J. D. A. (1997). *Disorders of affect regulation: Alexithymia in medical and psychiatric illness*. UK: Cambridge University Press

van der Hart, O., & Dorahy, M. J. (2009). History of the concept of dissociation. In P. F. Dell & J. A. O'Neil (Eds.), *Dissociation and the dissociative disorders: DSM-V and beyond* (pp. 3–26). London & New York: Routledge/Taylor & Francis Group.

Van der Hart, O., Nijenhuis, E. R. S., & Steele, K. (2006). *The haunted self: Structural dissociation and the treatment of chronic traumatization*. New York: W. W. Norton & Company.

Van der Hart, O. (2024). *Dissociazione da trauma*. Milano: Raffaello Cortina.

van der Kolk, B. A. (2014). *The body keeps the score: Brain, mind, and body in the healing of trauma*. London: Penguin Books.

Wiechelt, S. A., & Straussner, S. L. A. (Eds.). (2016). *Examining the relationship between trauma and addiction*. Routledge.

Wilson, S. J., Sayette, M. A., & Fiez, J. A. (2004). Prefrontal responses to drug cues: A neurocognitive analysis. *Nature Neuroscience*, 7, 211–214. doi:10.1038/nn1200.

Winhall, J. (2021). *Treating trauma and addiction with the felt sense polyvagal model: A bottom-up approach*. London & New York: Routledge.

Zagaria, A., Baggio, T., Rodella, L., & Leto, K. (2024). Toward a definition of attachment trauma: Integrating attachment and trauma studies. *European Journal of Trauma and Dissociation*, 8 (3), 1–16.

Zlotnick, C., Shea, M. T., Pearlstein, T., Begin, A., Simpson, E., & Costello, E. (1996). Differences in dissociative experiences between survivors of childhood incest and survivors of assault in adulthood. *Journal of Nervous and Mental Disease*, 184 (1), 52–54.

Index

Note: Locators in *italic* and **bold** refer figures and tables respectively, and locators followed by "n" refer end notes.